God's
Chosen
FAST

God's
Chosen
FAST

Arthur Wallis

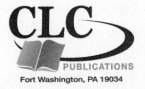
PUBLICATIONS
Fort Washington, PA 19034

Published by CLC Publications

U.S.A.
P.O. Box 1449, Fort Washington, PA 19034

GREAT BRITAIN
51 The Dean, Alresford, Hants SO24 9BJ

AUSTRALIA
P.O. Box 469, Kippa-Ring QLD 4021

NEW ZEALAND
118 King Street, Palmerston North 4410

Printed in the United States of America

ISBN-10: 0-87508-555-5
ISBN-13: 978-0-87508-555-5

Unless otherwise noted, Scripture quotations are from the Holy
Bible, Revised Standard Version, © 1946, 1952 by the Division
of Christian Education of the National Council of Churches of
Christ in the USA.

Italicized words in Scripture passages are the emphasis of the author.

The Scripture quotations in the diary are from the King James
Version.

Contents

Preface..7

1. Why Fast?..11

2. The Normal Fast...15

3. The Absolute Fast...19

4. The Partial Fast...23

5. "When"—Not "If"...27

6. The Time Is Now...29

7. The Regular and Public Fasts.............................35

8. Fasting unto God...41

9. For Personal Sanctity.......................................47

10. To Be Heard on High...53

11. To Change God's Mind.......................................59

12. To Free the Captives...63

13. They Fasted to Deliver......................................69

14. For Revelation...75

15. Fleshpots of Egypt...81

16. To Buffet the Body...87

17. What about Asceticism?....................................93

18. Fasting and the Body..99

19.   For Health and Healing...105

20.   How to Begin...111

21.   How to Break the Fast..115

22.   Diary of a Fast..121

23.   In the Last Days 133

      They Fasted 138

      Appendix I: Doubtful References to Fasting 141

      Appendix II: Answers to Practical Questions 145

      Appendix III: Healthy Eating..................................151

      Biblical Index 155

Preface

In a large city I inquired of all the Christian bookstores for some publication on the subject of fasting. They could not suggest a single title. A few days afterwards in a health food store in the same city, I picked up a book on health fasting. I soon discovered that there was far more being written on the physical aspect of this subject by food reformists than on the spiritual aspect by Christian writers. Later I was thankful to come across Gordon Cove's book *Revival Now Through Prayer and Fasting*, and a booklet by David Smith, *Some Light on Fasting*, containing helpful teaching and wise counsel. Apart from two or three American publications, there appeared to be nothing else in print.

Having proved the great value and blessing of fasting over many years, I was concerned that so many earnest believers had apparently never given the subject any serious thought. This concern became a constraint to share with those who hunger for God's best, what the Bible has to say about this spiritual exercise. My aim has been to furnish a handbook which would not only deal with the main passages in the Scripture that touch on the subject, including a biblical index, but to deal as fully as possible with the practical issues involved.

In the section of the book dealing with the physical and practical side, more space has been given to the longer fast, as a proper understanding of the physical aspect is so important. This should not lead the reader to suppose that everyone is called to undertake lengthy fasts, or that the shorter fast is of comparatively little value. This is by no means the case. Nevertheless, it is helpful for those who practice only the briefest fasting to understand the body's behavior in the longer fast.

Of course, the discussion of this physical side is the province of the physician rather than of the Bible student. Here I must record my indebtedness to the writings of Dr. Otto Buchinger of Germany and Dr. Herbert Shelton of San Antonio, Texas, both experts in the field of therapeutic fasting, as well as to those friends in the medical profession who kindly read the manuscript and carefully vetted what I have said on this side of the subject. I am most grateful to them and to others who have offered many helpful suggestions. I am also indebted to the late Professor James Orr for his article on asceticism in *The Protestant Dictionary*, and to the author of the article on fasting in *Hastings Encyclopaedia of Religion and Ethics*.

The neglect of truth followed by its rediscovery often results in its overemphasis. I have been aware of this temptation in connection with this subject and have therefore tried to give to this theme the weight that Scripture gives to it. Truth is like a portrait, and to exaggerate one feature is to turn the portrait into a caricature of the truth. The result is that thoughtful people turn from this divinely appointed means of grace as something for the crank or the fanatic.

Fasting *is* important—more important, perhaps, than many of us have supposed, as I trust this book will reveal. For all that, it is not a major biblical doctrine, a foundation stone of the faith, or a panacea for every spiritual ill. Nevertheless, when exercised with a pure heart and a right motive, fasting may provide us with a key to unlock doors where other keys have failed; a window opening up new horizons in the unseen world; a spiritual weapon of God's providing, "mighty, to the pulling down of strongholds." May God use this book to awaken many of His people to all the spiritual possibilities latent in the fast that God has chosen.

1

Why Fast?

For nearly a century and a half, fasting has been out of vogue, at least in the churches of the West. The very idea of someone actually fasting today seems strange to most twentieth-century Christians. They associate it with medieval Christianity, or perhaps with High Church practice. They may recall that political leaders, like Mahatma Ghandi, have used it as a weapon of passive resistance. As a spiritual exercise, it is confined, they would think, to believers who appear to be a little extreme or fanatical.

There are others whose misgivings concern the practical aspect. To them fasting and starving are synonymous terms, and they fear it will have harmful results. Because "no man ever hates his own flesh, but nourishes and cherishes it" (Eph. 5:29), they oppose fasting almost instinctively. "Do be careful," they say. "You could seriously impair your health. Living such a busy life you cannot afford to get run down!"

Why such attitudes to a practice that is so obviously scriptural? One answer is that fasting was one of the dominant features of an asceticism which began to appear in the post-apostolic age and became extreme in form as well as widespread in influence in medieval times. The pendulum began to swing the other way as people revolted against anything that savored of asceticism. The church today is still suffering from that reaction. We have not yet recovered the spiritual balance of New Testament Christianity.

The writer heard an able Bible teacher give a thought-provoking address on the reply our Lord gave to a question about fasting. It was that occasion when He said that the wedding guests would not fast until the Bridegroom was taken from them. All that the speaker said was most helpful, but he did not once touch upon the subject of fasting, or indicate whether it had any place in the economy of the Christian life today.

When our minds are conditioned by prejudice or para-lyzed by traditional views, we may face a truth in Scripture again and again without its ever touching us. Our spiritual inhibition concerning that truth permits us to see, but not to perceive. The truth lies dormant within, mentally ap-prehended but not spiritually applied. This is particularly true in relation to fasting.

When, however, such a truth is first ignited by the Holy Spirit, there is immediate conflict in the minds of most people. The truth of the Bible has suddenly become "alive and powerful," and there is an assault upon our traditional attitudes and prejudices.

The outcome of the struggle reveals whether or not we are open to receive and obey fresh light about God, and so grow in the knowledge of the truth. This book is intended to face us with the question of whether we are prepared to bring our present attitude about the subject of fasting (or our lack of one) to the acid test of God's Word, and then "live according to scripture" (1 Cor. 4:6).

Most of the references to fasting in the Bible are dealt with at some point in this book. It may surprise the reader, as it certainly did the writer, to find that Scripture has so much to teach us by example and by precept about the value of this practice. There are warnings too, for fasting has its dangers, and we have tried to point these out.

Among great Bible saints who fasted were Moses the lawgiver, David the king, Elijah the prophet and Daniel the seer. In the New Testament we have the example of our Lord as well as of His apostles. It clearly had its place in the life of the early churches. Nor was this biblical practice confined to men, for we find the names of Hannah in the Old Testament and Anna in the New Testament in the ranks of the intercessors who fasted as well as prayed.

Some of the great saints of church history have practiced fasting and testified to its value, among them the great Reformers, such as Luther, Calvin and Knox. The custom has not been confined to any theological school. Here we find Jonathan Edwards the Calvinist joining hands with John Wesley the Arminian, and David Brainerd having fellowship with Charles Finney.

These names represent great scholars and preachers, ministers and missionaries, revivalists and evangelists. We may find on the fasting list the names of Pastor Hsi of China and Pastor Blumhardt of Germany, whom God used in their respective spheres a century ago for the deliverance of those bound by Satan. Time would fail us to mention the growing number whom God is raising up and using in the same ministry today through prayer and fasting.

The doings of the great can scarcely be hidden. They are barely cold in their graves before their biographers are ferreting out their journals and private diaries. But only the opening of heaven's records in that day will reveal the numbers of anonymous saints, who had no diaries and no biographers, but who prayed with fasting to the God who sees in secret. They too shall surely shine among the galaxy of these illustrious saints, "even as the stars for ever and ever."

In New Testament times fasting was a channel of power. As spirituality waned and worldliness flourished in the churches, the power and gifts of the Spirit were withdrawn. With the loss of that inward power, men could only cling to what they had left, its outward accompaniment. More and more emphasis was placed upon the outward act of fasting, though bereft of the inward spirit that alone could give it value. Asceticism became the mark of piety and spirituality. Paul's prediction about "the form of religion but denying the power" (2 Tim. 3:5) was being fulfilled.

But, God be praised, a new day is dawning, and a new thirst for the Spirit is beginning to awaken the slumbering church. It is a day of spiritual renewal. There are searchings and inquirings, burdens and longings on every hand. The heart-cry of the church is ascending to heaven. The Spirit of God is stirring. What is all this but the first birthpangs of the new age that is soon to be born?

God is determined to have a glorious church without spot or wrinkle, a bride fit for His beloved Son. It is the conviction of the writer that, in the travail that will bring to birth, we shall rediscover one of the lost secrets of the early church: the power that is released through the truly biblical practice of fasting unto God.

2

The Normal Fast

He fasted forty days and forty nights and afterward he was hungry. Matthew 4:2

When people do not like the plain, literal meaning of something in the Bible, they are tempted to spiritualize it and so rob it of its potency. Once the truth becomes nebulous, it ceases to have any practical application. They have blunted its edge; it can no longer cut. In the main this is what the professing church, and evangelicals in particular, have tended to do with the biblical teaching on fasting.

"To fast," we are told, "is not simply nor necessarily to abstain from food, but from anything that hinders our communion with God." Or they say, "Fasting means to do without, to practice self-denial." We have only to widen the meaning enough, and the cutting edge has gone.

It is true that there are many things besides food that may hinder our communion with God. It is also true that we need to practice self-denial in general. The fact still remains that "to fast" means primarily "not to eat."[1] We shall see that there were three main forms that fasting took in Bible times, but each involved literal abstinence. If at times the word may be widened to include other forms of self-denial, this does not alter the fact of its basic meaning.

For convenience sake let us call this first and most common form *the normal fast*. What this involved is plain from the first mention of fasting in the New Testament: Jesus fasted . . . and afterwards He was hungry. It meant abstaining from all food, solid or liquid, but not from water. It seems clear from the details given that our Lord's fast was of this type.

We are told that "he ate nothing" (Luke 4:2), but not that He drank nothing. Afterward it says "he was hungry," but not that He was thirsty. Though thirst pangs are more intense than those of hunger, Satan tempted Him to eat, but not to drink. This all suggests that the fast was an abstaining from food, but not from water. In fact, the human body could not survive forty days without water apart from being supernaturally sustained.

There is nothing to suggest that true fasting involves abstaining from sleep. God may call us to do this for very short periods, such as giving up a night's sleep. Paul speaks of "watchings" as distinct from "fastings" (2 Cor. 6:5; 11:27, KJV.). If abstaining from sleep was essential to fasting, no long fast would ever be possible apart from supernatural intervention. The body craves sleep even before water and is bound to succumb sooner or later, and the fast will be broken involuntarily.

There is a strong inference in First Corinthians 7:3–5 that the true fast for married persons includes abstaining also from marital relations, but this must be by mutual consent. We cannot be dogmatic here, as it seems certain that the inclusion of the word "fasting" (7:5) in the text of the King James Version is a gloss and no part of the original.[2] Nevertheless, the idea of fasting is there.

The normal fast, then, involved abstaining from all forms of food, but not from water, and must be distinguished from the other two forms, *the absolute fast* and t*he partial fast*, which we must now consider.

1. Greek *nesteuo*, from *ne*, a negative prefix, and *esthio*, "to eat."
2. See Appendix I.

3

The Absolute Fast

For three days he . . . neither ate nor drank. Acts 9:9

We have a few examples in Scripture of what we have called the absolute fast, that is, abstaining from drinking as well as eating. Normally this was never for more than three days, probably because any longer period might have proved physically injurious. The body can go long periods without food and be physically benefited, but only for a very short time without water.

We read of Ezra that "he spent the night, neither eating bread nor drinking water; for he was mourning over the faithlessness of the exiles" (Ezra 10:6). He was overcome with grief and astonishment at the shameful compromise of the people in which priests, Levites and officials had given the lead. He says, "I rent my garments and my mantle, and pulled hair from my head and beard, and sat appalled" (9:3). Overwhelming concern drove him to fast, taking neither food nor water.

Queen Esther instructed Mordecai, "Hold a fast on my behalf, and neither eat nor drink for three days, night or day. I and my maids will also fast as you do" (Esther 4:16). A crisis of the utmost gravity threatened the whole Jewish race with extermination. Even Esther herself could expect no immunity because she was queen. She called this absolute fast because desperate situations require desperate measures.

Saul of Tarsus arrived in Damascus dazed and blinded by his encounter with the risen Christ. "And for three days he . . . neither ate nor drank" (Acts 9:9). The spiritual revolution that was taking place within the young Pharisee was not only to alter the whole course of his life but to shape the history of the Christian church. Possibly the upheaval was so great that he never gave food or drink a thought.

There are examples in Scripture of absolute fasts which must have been supernatural in character because of their very long duration. For two separate periods of forty days and forty nights, Moses was in the presence of God, neither eating nor drinking (Deut. 9:9,18; Exod. 34:28). The first occasion was when he received the Ten Commandments from God. The second was immediately following, after discovering the people were worshipping the golden calf and so had broken the law even before they had formally received it. These two fasts were undertaken virtually without intermission, and taken together constitute what is certainly the longest fast in the Bible, eighty days without food or water.

Then the journey of Elijah to Horeb appears to have been undertaken during an absolute fast. If so, it must have been supernatural. Under the juniper tree, where he was sleeping after escaping from Jezebel, he was awakened by an angel who provided him with a freshly baked cake and a cruse of water. Twice he was told to eat and drink, and then he "went in the strength of that food forty days and forty nights to Horeb the mount of God" (1 Kings 19:8).

A journey of such duration through the burning desert, if it was completed, as the Scripture implies, without further nourishment, constitutes an absolute fast quite as supernatural as those of Moses. If that be so, it is another striking parallel between these two leading representatives of the old covenant, Moses the giver of the Law and Elijah its restorer (Mal. 4:4–6; Mark 9:12), for both had a supernatural ending to their earthly course as well as a supernatural reappearance with Christ on the holy mount.

Leaving aside such fasts as these which were epoch-making and supernatural, we conclude that the absolute fast is an exceptional measure for an exceptional situation. It is something usually reserved for spiritual emergencies. One knows of extreme cases of need which have not yielded to normal prayer and fasting, but which have responded when the intercessor was led by God to fast absolutely. This is especially true in cases of powerful possession by evil spirits. One would need to be very sure of the leading of God to undertake such a fast for any period longer than three days.

4

The Partial Fast

I ate no delicacies, no meat or wine entered my mouth.
Daniel 10:3

The emphasis here is upon restriction of diet rather than complete abstention. At the commencement of the book of Daniel, we are introduced to this young man and his three companions. They had been selected from among the Hebrew exiles because of noble birth and intellectual attainments for special training, with a view to serving in the presence of the king of Babylon.

These men resolved not to defile themselves with the king's rich food or the wine which he drank, as these would have been first offered to the Babylonian gods. Instead, they asked for vegetables to eat and water to drink. The steward set over them agreed to test the effect of this simple diet for a period of ten days. At the end of this time, "they were better in appearance and fatter in flesh than all the youths who ate the king's rich food" (Dan. 1:15).

Whether or not there was supernatural intervention here is difficult to tell, but it is a commonly accepted fact of dietetics that a simple and wholesome diet is far more beneficial than a rich and elaborate one. Those who move in a circle where there is constant dining and wining are often beset with ailments caused by excess, including coronary thrombosis. All forms of fasting, on the other hand, are physically beneficial, and many who are outside Christian circles fast for health reasons alone.

The value of the partial fast, however, is not confined by any means to the physical. Later in the book of Daniel, we read how this prophet received a revelation from God concerning the future of his people Israel. He describes how he sought the Lord for understanding of this vision: "In those days I, Daniel, was mourning for three weeks. I ate no delicacies, no meat or wine entered my mouth, nor did I anoint myself at all, for the full three weeks" (Dan. 10:2–3).

We are not told why he did not engage in a normal fast, as we find him doing in the previous chapter. Possibly affairs of state or other circumstances precluded this; or perhaps it was simply that God guided him otherwise. Undoubtedly there is a definite spiritual value in a special season of seeking God with such a restricted diet. For Daniel it resulted in a great spiritual victory over the powers of darkness as well as the unfolding of the vision by an angelic messenger.

Something akin to a partial fast is seen in the period of Elijah's spiritual preparation. At Cherith the raven brought him bread and meat morning and evening, and he drank from the brook. Later in the home of the widow at Zarephath, he was sustained with simple cakes made from meal and oil (1 Kings 17).

Besides the training of this man of God in self-denial, indispensable to one who is to be entrusted with spiritual power, it was appropriate that the diet of God's servant should be the simplest while there was a famine in the land, and many of his fellow countrymen were facing starvation. To minister effectively to those in need, we must be identified with their need and sit where they sit.

A Russian believer deeply impressed a Christian couple when she went to stay on their farm in England a few years ago. Miraculously converted, she had been called by God to work for Him in a displaced persons camp in Austria. She politely declined the Cornish cream which made its appearance at almost every meal, and permitted herself only the simplest diet, explaining that she could not do otherwise when her brothers, sisters and those among whom she labored were enduring such hardship. God never fails to honor such self-denial.

Elijah's counterpart in the New Testament was John the Baptist. We learn from the gospel records that in addition to fasting often, he maintained the simplest of diets, subsisting on locusts and wild honey.

The partial fast allows a great many variations which have been tried with blessing and benefit. There is the method of living exclusively on one type of food for the duration of the fast. During his early days in Georgia, John Wesley adopted a "bread diet," that is, living exclusively on dry bread. This was in connection with what he believed was a case of demon-possession.[1]

Others have partially fasted by omitting a certain meal each day, thus strictly limiting the quantity of food consumed. We learn from his biography that Rees Howells adopted this plan at a time when God was preparing him for a new work: "He didn't take dinner for many days . . . but spent the hour with God."[2] Vigilance is needed to ensure that the value of omitting the one meal is not offset by increasing the intake at others!

The partial fast is of great value, especially where circumstances make it impossible or inconvenient to undertake a normal fast. Certainly it requires no less self-discipline. It can be used as a steppingstone to the normal fast by those

who have never fasted before. One of its great advantages
is that even after being sustained for a long period, normal
eating can be resumed almost at once, which is not the case
with the other two kinds of fasting.

Later we shall notice that under these three main fasts
we have now considered, biblical fasting may be public as
well as private, regular as well as occasional, involuntary as
well as voluntary. We shall notice too the differing needs
and circumstances that moved men to fast, and their application for us today. But first let us examine the two key
statements of our Lord on fasting, for these must determine
our attitude to the whole subject.

1. N. Churnock, ed., *Wesley's Journals*, Vol. I.
2. Norman Grubb, *Rees Howells, Intercessor*. CLC Publications.

5

"When"—Not "If"

When you give alms . . . when you pray . . . when you fast.
Matthew 6:2, 5, 16

In the great commission Christ commanded His apostles, "Make disciples of all nations . . . teaching them to observe all that I have commanded you" (Matt. 28:19–20). There has been for a century or more a tendency to emphasize and elevate the teaching of the Epistles in such a way as to suggest that it supersedes the teaching of Christ as we have it in the Gospels.

Some have even asserted that the teaching of the Sermon on the Mount has no direct application to believers today, that it is basically Messianic and Jewish, to be fulfilled in some future millennial age. This is serious error, and in direct conflict with Christ's commission just quoted. If these words have any meaning, it is surely that what Jesus taught His disciples was to be taught to every successive generation of disciples, and obeyed, even to the consummation of the age (see also 1 Tim. 6:3–4).

What did our Lord teach His disciples concerning fasting? That must surely rule our conduct now. Quoted above is the first of His two vital utterances on this subject.

In speaking about giving, praying and fasting, Jesus

warned His hearers of the futility of practicing their piety before men to be seen by them (Matt. 6:1–18). He did not say, "*If* you pray," as though praying were optional, but, "*When* you pray," taking for granted that they would recognize prayer as a vital necessity.

Neither did Jesus say, "*If* you fast," as though fasting were something that disciples might or might not be led to do, or as though it only applied to a select few, apostles or prophets, preachers or leaders. He stated unambiguously, categorically and without qualification to the mass of His disciples, "*When* you fast . . . ." He left us in no doubt that He took it for granted that His disciples would be exercised to obey the leading of the Spirit in this, as in praying and giving, when the occasion demanded it.

It is significant that the Lord dealt with fasting as a spiritual exercise distinct from praying. Though fasting and praying are often linked in Scripture and in experience, this is not necessarily the case. We should not think of fasting as a semi-detached house, always joined to praying. On the contrary, it stands on its own grounds and may on occasion serve a spiritual purpose all its own.

Just as there may be praying without fasting, so there may at times be fasting, truly acceptable to God, without praying—at least in the sense of intercession. There is no mention of prayer accompanying the fast we read of in Esther. In the fast of the prophets and teachers in Antioch, they were giving themselves to worship rather than prayer (Acts 13:2).

Because one is not able to give oneself to prayer for the whole of a fast does not mean that the period not accompanied by specific prayer is devoid of spiritual value. Fasting, as we shall notice later, has many purposes besides the very important one of facilitating intercession.

6

The Time Is Now

*When the bridegroom is taken from them . . . then
they will fast.* Matthew 9:15

This second important statement of Jesus on fasting
came as an answer to a question of the disciples of John
the Baptist: "Why," they asked, "do we and the Pharisees
fast, but your disciples do not fast?" Christ's answer is deeply
pertinent to the question of whether Christians should fast
today. He said, "Can the wedding guests mourn as long as
the bridegroom is with them? The days will come when
the bridegroom is taken away from them, and then they
will fast."

Though there were times when Jesus and His disciples
went hungry or when, due to the demands of the work,
they had not sufficient leisure to eat, there is no evidence
that He or they undertook a definite voluntary fast, other
than our Lord's forty days in the wilderness prior to the
commencement of His public ministry. Here He gives the
reason: the bridegroom was still with the wedding guests.

It was a season of feasting not fasting, of rejoicing not
mourning. A new day had dawned. The kingdom of God
had drawn near. The old order with its rites and ceremonies
and legal bondage had gone forever. Even when the Bride-

groom was taken from them, there would be no return to the legalism and asceticism of the old order. Though His disciples would fast again, it would be for different reasons and in a different spirit from that which characterized the fasting of the Pharisees, or even of John the Baptist. As Jesus went on to explain, the old Judaistic wineskin was not a suitable receptacle for the new wine of the Spirit.

"The days will come when the bridegroom is taken away from them, and then they will fast." This is perhaps the most crucial statement in the New Testament on the question of fasting. To what period of time was Jesus referring? Could He have meant the very brief period following His arrest, until He reappeared in resurrection? Some have thought so from His words, "A little while, and you will see me no more; again a little while, and you will see me. . . . Truly, truly, I say to you, you will weep and lament, but the world will rejoice; you will be sorrowful, but your sorrow will turn into joy" (John 16:16, 20). The view has been expressed thus:

> He was taken away from them, and they fasted and were sad through those days of darkness; but He came back, and, standing on the slope of Olivet, He said, "Lo, I am with you alway." Then there is no more room for mourning; no more room for the sad face of agony; but there is room for mirth, room for joy, and room for gladness.[1]

According to this view, the days of the absent Bridegroom were limited to three or at the most four. With Christ's resurrection and reappearance, the period of fasting has passed away.

Very pleasant as it may be to hold this view, it would seem to be untenable for several reasons. Firstly, this age is not one of undiminished joy. Joy there certainly is, but it is not unmixed with sadness. There is surely room for mourning while sin and sorrow and conflict are all around us. "We must through many tribulations enter the kingdom of God."

Apart from all this, how could there be unclouded joy while our beloved Lord and Master is still waiting to receive His kingdom, to see of the travail of His soul and be satisfied? Surely His own words, "Blessed are they that mourn," must have application to this age.

Then again the Lord's words stress only two periods of time. There was the time of joy, "as long as the bridegroom is with them," which was then being fulfilled. There was the time of sorrow to follow: "The days will come, when the bridegroom is taken away from them." But the above interpretation puts the emphasis on a third phrase, when the Bridegroom came back to them, which is not in view in this statement of Christ.

In our Lord's analogy the guests at the wedding rejoice because the bridegroom is with them. The festivities over, the bridegroom departs, and the guests are sad because they do no know when they will see him again. "The days will come, when the bridegroom is taken away from them" suggests an absence of unspecified duration, but surely longer than the brief spell of the festivities.

The time of joy and feasting clearly represents the years of His earthly ministry. Is it likely that the time of mourning and fasting could have been fulfilled in those few days of absence before He appeared in resurrection? And, in any case, where is the evidence that they fasted during those three days? When He appeared to them in the upper room and asked them if they had anything to eat, they were able to produce a piece of fish ready cooked (Luke 24:41–42).

We are therefore compelled to refer the days of His absence to the period of this age, from the time He ascended to the Father until He shall return from heaven. This is evidently how His apostles understood Him, for it was not until after His ascension to the Father that we read of them fasting (Acts 13:2–3).

Before the Bridegroom left them He promised that He would come again to receive them unto Himself. The church still awaits the midnight cry, "Behold, the bridegroom! Come out to meet him" (Matt. 25:6). It is this age of the church that is the period of the absent Bridegroom. It is this age of the church to which our Master referred when He said, "*Then* they will fast." The time is *now*!

These words of Jesus were prophetic. The first Christians fulfilled them, and so have many saintly men and women of suceeding generations. Where are those who fulfill them today? Alas, they are few and far between, the exception rather than the rule, to the great loss of the church.

A new generation, however, is arising. There is concern in the hearts of many for the recovery of apostolic power. But how can we recover apostolic power while neglecting apostolic practice? How can we expect the power to flow if we do not prepare the channels? Fasting is a God-appointed means for the flowing of His grace and power that we can afford to neglect no longer.

The fast of this age is not merely an act of mourning for Christ's absence, but an act of preparation for His return. May those prophetic words "Then will they fast" be finally fulfilled in this generation. It will be a fasting and praying church that will hear the thrilling cry, "Behold, the Bridegroom!" Tears shall then be wiped away, and *the fast* be followed by *the feast* at the marriage supper of the Lamb.

> The Spirit and the Bride say, "Come."
> "Surely I am coming soon."
> Amen. Come, Lord Jesus! (Rev. 22:17, 20)

1. G. Campbell Morgan, *The Gospel According to Matthew*, Fleming H. Revell Co.

7

The Regular and Public Fasts

On a fast day . . . you shall read the words of the Lord.
Jeremiah 36:6

Sanctify a fast; call a solemn assembly. Joel 2:15

We have already noted that normally fasting is undertaken occasionally, as the need arises, and that it is a personal matter between the individual and God. The *regular* and *public* fasts, of which Scripture gives a number of examples, are obvious exceptions. There is a connection between these two in that almost all the regular fasts of the Bible were also public ones, but not all the public ones were necessarily regular.

The Day of Atonement, on which God had said that every Israelite was to afflict himself (Lev. 23:27; see also Ps. 35:13 and Isa. 58:5, KJV), was the only regular fast prescribed by the Mosaic Law. From Acts 27:9 we learn that this fast was still observed by Jews in New Testament times. In addition to "a fast day" in the time of Jeremiah quoted above, we find in Zechariah 8:19 four regular fasts commemorating the four main events connected with the destruction of Jerusalem.[1]

By the time of Christ, the Pharisees had developed this practice of regular fasting and had turned it, like every other spiritual thing they touched, into a legal bondage. Thus, Christ presents us with a picture of the typical Pharisee as a man who boasts in his prayer, "I fast twice a week" (Luke 18:11–12). In the second and third centuries after Christ, the Wednesday and Friday of each week became recognized as fast days, and John Wesley revived this custom among the early Methodists.

There is always the danger that any spiritual exercise that is done habitually becomes an empty form, a ritual devoid of any spiritual content. But we cannot reject the practice of regular fasting on account of this danger. We do not abandon regular seasons of prayer or the habit of giving regularly to God because the Pharisees abused these also. Regular fasting need not become ritualistic, any more than regular praying.

It needs to be stressed that fasting, whether regular or occasional, is a matter between the individual and God. The lessons of history would teach us to resist any tendency to allow regular fasting by the individual to become a church custom. One short step and the church custom has become a church rule to which the faithful are obliged to bow, and another yoke has been placed upon the neck of the disciples which neither the church fathers nor their successors were able to bear. More will be said about this in the chapter on asceticism.

Provided we watch these dangers and see to it that the habit does not become a form devoid of spirit and life, and that we do not try to force our personal exercise of heart upon others, there is real value in the regular fast. Not only does it provide a regular opportunity for spiritual examination and reorientation, but it is also a valuable means of conserving that increasingly precious commodity called "time." A regular fast one day a week could mean that the time spent over three meals, say two hours, is reclaimed from our busy program and invested more specifically in the kingdom of God, especially in the great ministry of prayer. Here is a weekly tonic for both soul and body, which could also be an instrument for the blessing of others.

Among those who permitted themselves to indulge in this luxury, mention might be made of that patriarch of the Open Brethren, Robert Chapman of Barnstaple (1803–1902). It was his custom to spend every Saturday fasting. He did not see visitors on this day, but shut himself up in his workshop, alone with God and with his lathe—a time of recreation, communion, as well as preparation of his soul for the coming Lord's Day. It is recorded that someone who had to make an emergency visit to the workshop one Saturday said, "His face shone as the face of an angel."[2]

Who can tell how much this practice contributed to the spiritual stature that Robert Chapman attained and the rare intimacy of his walk with God? Many would desire to attain to his sanctity of heart and life without a willingness to tread the path he trod. "Why are we not more holy?" asked John Wesley, another regular faster, addressing his preachers. "Chiefly because we are enthusiasts, looking for the end without the means."

These regular fasts of the Old Testament were both national and public. But there were also public fasts that were not regular, but confined to times of special need and emergency. King Jehoshaphat called the nation to fast when Judah was invaded (2 Chron. 20:1–4), and Ezra likewise exhorted the returning exiles, before their perilous journey back to Jerusalem with the precious things for the temple (Ezra 8:21–23). Most spectacular of all was the public fast undertaken by the city of Nineveh as a result of Jonah's preaching, which we shall consider in a later chapter.

These and other instances reveal that the public fast was called for in times of national or spiritual crisis, in much the same way as in the Second World War the King called the British to a day of prayer. Two centuries earlier, the same nation was called to "a day of solemn fasting and prayer" in view of a threatened invasion by the French. On Friday, February 6, 1756, Wesley records in his journals:

> The fast day was a glorious day, such as London has scarce seen since the Restoration. Every church in the city was more than full, and a solemn seriousness sat on every face. Surely God heareth prayer, and there will yet be a lengthening of our tranquillity.

A footnote informs us:

> Humility was turned into national rejoicing for the threatened invasion by the French was averted.

Wherever in Scripture we read of a public emergency being met by a national call to fast, we find without exception that God responded in deliverance. As grave national and international crises undoubtedly lie ahead, it would be well for us to remember this ancient biblical practice of sanctifying a public fast. Even if only the godly within the nation are ready to respond, they will find that God's promise holds good: "I will hear from heaven, and will forgive their sin and heal their land" (2 Chron. 7:14).

If there is a local church threatened with discord and division, if spiritual life is waning and worldliness abounding, if conversions are few and backslidings frequent, would not this be a time when leaders should call that church to prayer and fasting?

Before leaving this section we should observe that fasting may also refer in Scripture to abstaining from food involuntarily. The two kinds of involuntary fasting are where there is no desire for food because of anxiety, sorrow or mental distress (Dan. 6:18), and where persons find themselves in a situation where no food is available (Matt. 15:32).

Paul evidently knew a good deal of this latter sort. Some commentators take his mention of "fastings" in Second Corinthians 6:5 and 11:27 to refer to this kind of involuntary hardship, as the Revised Standard Version rendering here confirms. Evidently Paul had no difficulty in reconciling such experiences of want with the promise, "My God will supply every need of yours." He knew that the experience of finding himself temporarily without food, and without the means to obtain it, was a necessary trial of faith permitted by God for his ultimate blessing. In the very context of the wonderful promise, he says: "I have learned, in whatever state I am, to be content. I know how to be abased, and I know how to abound; in any and all circumstances I have learned the secret of facing plenty and hunger, abundance and want" (Phil. 4:11–12).

If God should even call us to walk for a moment "the path of necessity," and we find ourselves on a fast that is not our choosing, let us not fear. He will yet turn our captivity and bless our latter end more than our beginning.

1. Tenth month, beginning of the siege (2 Kings 25:1). Fourth month, fall of the city (Jer. 39:2). Fifth month, destruction of city and temple (2 Kings 25:8–9). Seventh month, murder of Gedaliah (2 Kings 25:25).
2. Frank Holmes, *Brother Indeed*. Victory Press.

8

Fasting unto God

When ye fasted . . . did ye at all fast unto me, even to me? Zechariah 7:5

They ministered to the Lord, and fasted. Acts 13:2

Fasting today! Whatever is to be gained by that?" is the incredulous question of many Christians. If they mean, "What does one personally gain by fasting?" then there are many answers that may be given, and will be given in this book, but there is a more important question to answer first.

So much of our thinking is ruled by that self-centered principle, "What do I get out of it?" Even in our spiritual desires and aspirations, self may still be enthroned. The cross must work in us if the life is to be centered in God. Only so can our spiritual motivation be radically altered and become Christward instead of self-ward. "He died for all, that they which live should no longer live unto themselves, but unto him" (2 Cor. 5:15, RV).

Even in circles where fasting is accepted as a normal spiritual exercise, there is often so much emphasis on fasting for personal benefit, for the enduement of power, for spiritual gifts, for physical healing, for specific answers to prayer, that the other aspect is forgotten. There is no suggestion that it is not right to seek these things, but our underlying motives must first be right. It is deeply significant that in the first statement on the subject of fasting in the New Testament, Jesus dealt with the question of motive (Matt. 6:16–18). No aspect of the subject is more important than this.

God is not merely concerned with what we do but why we do it. A right act may be robbed of all its value in the sight of God if it is done with a wrong motive. The danger of this is acute in the realm of outward religious exercises. "Why have we fasted, and thou seest it not?" asked the perplexed religionists of Isaiah's day. Swift was heaven's answer, "Behold, in the day of your fast you seek your own pleasure" (Isa. 58:3). The fasts they undertook, with all their show of piety, were motivated by self-interest and self-seeking. No wonder God asked indignantly, "Is such the fast that I choose?" (58:5).

This same self-centerness under a cloak of piety was seen in all its shameful hypocrisy in the fasting of the Pharisees, and it was against this that Jesus lifted up His voice in the Sermon on the Mount, telling His followers that when they fasted they were not to be like the hypocrites. The Pharisees paraded their piety for the applause of men by making sure that people knew they were fasting. They were not ministering to God but to the pride of their own hearts. Later, when Jesus described the Pharisee praying in the temple and saying, "God, I thank thee that I am not like other men. . . . I fast twice a week," He is careful to inform us that he "prayed thus with himself" (Luke 18:11–12).

Fasting must be done unto God, even before the eye of the Father who sees in secret. While avoiding the brazen conceit of the Pharisee and the desire to court the praise of man, we may still act out of selfish motives, for the gratification of personal desires and ambitions, and without the basic motive being the glory of God.

In Isaiah 58, the classic of Scripture on the subject of fasting, God reminds His people that the acceptable fast is the one which *He* has chosen. Fasting, like prayer, must be God-initiated and God-ordained if it is to be effective. Prevailing prayer begins with God; He places upon us a burden by the Spirit, and we respond to that burden. Prayer that originates with God always returns to God. So it is with fasting. When God chooses our fast, He will not have to ask us, as He asked His people long ago, "When ye fasted . . . did ye at all fast unto me, even to me?" (Zech. 7:5, RV).

All this does not of course relieve us of our responsibility. On our part there must be the recognition of the rightness and need of fasting, the willingness for the self-discipline involved, and the exercise of heart before God; but in the final analysis the initiative is His. When we fast, how long we fast, the nature of the fast and the spiritual objectives we have before us are all God's choice, to which the obedient disciple gladly responds.

This principle applies even to *the regular fast*, say one day a week. We must be sure that God is leading us to do this. Even then there may be times when it will be inconvenient to carry it out, or when we are guided not to do so; or a time may come when we are led to discontinue the practice. We are not to be in bondage to rules, even spiritual ones. "If you are led by the Spirit you are not under the law" (Gal. 5:18). When Joel cried, "Sanctify a fast," he meant "Set it apart for God." This is absolutely basic if our fasting is to be acceptable to Him. Then there will be times when we shall forget the matter of our personal gain, when we shall be caught up in wonder, love and praise, as we fast unto God. We shall find ourselves like Anna the prophetess, "worshipping with fasting" (Luke 2:37), or like those leaders of the church in Antioch who "ministered to the Lord, and fasted" (Acts 13:2, KJV; "worshipping the Lord," RSV). This is surely the loftiest conception, that it is a worshipping or ministering to the Lord, a giving of ourselves to God, and only secondarily a means to secure certain spiritual ends.

We cannot do better than to quote in conclusion from John Wesley's famous sermon on fasting:

> First, let it be done unto the Lord, with our eye singly fixed on Him. Let our intention herein be this, and this alone, to glorify our Father which is in heaven; to express our sorrow and shame for our manifold transgressions of His holy law; to wait for an increase of purifying grace, drawing our affections to things above; to add seriousness and to obtain all the great and precious promises which He hath made to us in Jesus Christ. . . . Let us beware of fancying we *merit* anything of God by our fasting. We cannot be too often warned of this; inasmuch as a desire to "establish our own righteousness," to procure salvation of debt and not of grace, is so deeply rooted in all our hearts. Fasting is only a way which God hath ordained, wherein we wait for His unmerited mercy; and wherein, without any desert of ours, He hath promised freely to give us His blessing.[1]

God's chosen fast, then, is that which He has appointed; that which is set apart for Him, to minister to Him, to honor and glorify Him; that which is designed to accomplish His sovereign will. Then we shall find, as though it were heaven's afterthought, that the fast unto God rebounds in blessing on our heads, and the God who sees in secret is graciously pleased to reward us openly. In this way we are preserved from ever permitting the blessings to mean more to us than the Blesser, "For from Him and through

Him and to Him are all things. To Him be glory for ever. Amen" (Rom. 11:36).

1. John Wesley, *Sermon 27* (Discourse 7 on the Sermon on the Mount, Matt. 6:16–18).

9

For Personal Sanctity

I humbled my soul with fasting. Psalm 69:10

Blessed are those who mourn. Matthew 5:4

We have now seen what fasting is. We have established that it is a biblical practice, and that it is for today. We have distinguished various types of fasts and seen how essential it is that our motives are right: that we fast unto God. Now we come to examine in Scripture the purposes of fasting. Here, then, is the first answer to the question, "What is the good of it?" It is a valuable aid to personal sanctity.

If humility is the basic ingredient of true holiness, the soil in which the graces flourish, is it not needful that from time to time we should, like David, humble our souls with fasting? Behind many of our besetting sins and personal failures, behind the many ills that infect our church fellowships and clog the channels of Christian service—the clash of personalities and temperaments, the strife and division—lies that insidious pride of the human heart.

How is it that fasting can help us here? On the negative side pride and a too-full stomach are old bedfellows. What was the sin of Sodom? Not primarily that gross form of immorality known anciently as sodomy, now called homosexuality. The Bible says, "This was the guilt of your

sister Sodom, pride, surfeit of food, and prosperous ease"
(Ezek. 16:49).

When we look at the nations of the West today where
this sin of Sodom is rampant, we can discern the same root
causes. History cannot help repeating itself. Given the same
conditions, the same malaise inevitably follows.

God foresaw that pride and full feeding would be one
of Israel's pitfalls when they entered the land of promise.
"God has led you these forty years in the wilderness," Moses
reminded them. "He humbled you and let you hunger."
(Deut. 8:2–3). Now those days of discipline were over, and
the land of plenty that they were about to possess would
provide new temptations, so Moses went on to warn them,
"Take heed . . . lest, when you have eaten and are full . . .
your heart be lifted up" (8:11–14). Hosea tells us that this
is exactly what happened (Hos. 13:6), despite the warning.

Fasting, then, is a divine corrective to the pride of the
human heart. It is a discipline of the body with a tendency
to humble the soul. "I proclaimed a fast there, at the river
Ahava, that we might humble ourselves before our God,"
records Ezra (8:21; see also Isa. 58:3).

If, then, to the devout Israelite fasting meant humbling,
it also meant mourning. In fact, in Old Testament days it
was practiced as a sign of mourning for the departed, almost
as a part of the funeral rites (1 Sam. 31:13, etc.). It is associated with the rending of the garment and the wearing
of sackcloth and ashes (Ezra 9:5, etc.). In Matthew 9:15
we have seen how our Lord treated "mourn" and "fast" as
interchangeable terms.

There is a natural sequence as we move from self-
humbling to the mourning of repentance and contrition.
Israel fasted in repentance in the days of Samuel, and so did
the returned exiles in the time of Nehemiah (1 Sam. 7:6;

Neh. 9:1–2). Mourning over personal sin and failure is an indispensable stage in the process of sanctification, and it is facilitated by fasting.

However, God wants to bring us beyond the place of mourning only for our personal sins, to where we are moved by the Spirit to mourn for the sins of the church, the nation, and even the world. It is of the deepest concern to God to find those who share His feelings for the spiritual situation that exists on every hand.

Ezekiel was given a vision of the judgment of God coming upon Jerusalem because of its abominations. Before the heavenly executioners were permitted to destroy the inhabitants of the city, a man was sent before them to "put a mark upon the foreheads of the men who sigh and groan over all the abominations that are committed in it." The executioners were then commanded to go forth and slay without mercy all except those who had the mark, and to begin at God's sanctuary (Ezek. 9:4–6).

Heaven marks the men who feel with God for the sins that break His heart and turn away His face from us. The same abominations are still being committed in sanctuary and in city. If today God put a mark on those who sigh and groan because of this, and then sent forth His executioners to destroy all but those with the mark, would we escape?

Will such mourning accomplish anything? Indeed, it may be just as remedial in the corporate sphere as in the personal. True, in Ezekiel's vision the sin of the people had reached the point of "no return," and judgment had become inevitable, but this is by no means always the case. There is always the hope that spiritual forces will be released which will work toward repentance and recovery.

The eyes of the Lord are still searching the earth today for the Ezras who will confess the sins of a faithless remnant, weeping and casting themselves down before the Lord; or the Nehemiahs who will weep and mourn, fast and pray for the walls that are broken down, and the gates that are destroyed by fire. If restoration and renewal are to come from the presence of the Lord—and what hope is there without them?—then it is men and women like these whom God will use to turn the tide.

In the fasting for personal sanctity, we must also include the positive aspect of *consecration to God*. Perhaps the best example of this is the forty day fast undertaken by our Lord prior to His public ministry. His baptism in the Jordan was His dedication unto death in anticipation of the cross. Though He received the Spirit then in measureless fullness, the power was not operative until He returned from the wilderness testing. By His acceptance of those six weeks of fasting, He was reaffirming His determination to do the will of His Father even to the end. It was His final preparation and consecration for His heavenly mission. As He returned to Galilee in the power of the Spirit, the works of God were manifested in Him.

Something of this is seen in the setting apart of Barnabas and Paul for their apostolic ministry. "Then after fasting and praying they laid their hands on them and sent them off" (Acts 13:3). Not a social tea but a consecration fast marked the first missionary valedictory. Later we see these men appointing elders in every church, with prayer and fasting (Acts 14:23). Thus were the local leaders consecrated to their holy office. Where are the churches today where the leaders are set apart in a solemn season of prayer and fasting? Perhaps here is one reason why office in the church is so often lightly taken up, loosely held and readily tossed aside when difficulties or differences emerge. Little wonder we lack strong spiritual leadership, and the sheep tend to drift.

If you have been brought low through personal defeat; if there is a call in your soul to a deeper purifying, to a renewed consecration; if there is the challenge of some new task for which you feel ill-equipped—then it is time to inquire of God whether He would not have you separate yourself unto Him in fasting.

10

To Be Heard on High

So we fasted and besought our God for this,
and he listened to our entreaty. Ezra 8:23

Isaiah lived in a day when formalism and hypocrisy had rendered the religious exercise of fasting obnoxious to God. But we need to remember that this was also true of their offerings, their prayers and their worship (Isa. 1:10–15). In that remarkable chapter on fasting, Isaiah 58, God not only uncovered the self-seeking and self-pleasing which lay behind this show of piety, but He went on to unfold the character of the fast that He *had* chosen, and the blessing that it could bring to others as well as themselves.

Fasting is here connected with seeking God, drawing near to God, prevailing with God. These ends, however, were not being realized, because their motive in fasting was not a right one. God had to say: "Fasting like yours this day will not make your voice to be heard on high" (58:4). But that is clearly one thing that fasting is intended to do, for, describing the fast that He has chosen, God goes on to say, "Then you shall call and the Lord will answer" (58:9).

Fasting is designed to make prayer mount up as on eagles' wings. It is intended to usher the suppliant into the audience chamber of the King and to extend to him the golden sceptre. It may be expected to drive back the oppressing powers of darkness and loosen their hold on the prayer objective. It is calculated to give an edge to a man's intercessions and power to his petitions. Heaven is ready to bend its ear to listen when someone prays with fasting.

How often we have made earnest prayer to God for some specific need, with the assurance that this was in the will of God, and yet there has been no answer from heaven. Why? It could well be, and often is, that God is saying to us, "When you seek me *with all your heart*, I will be found by you" (Jer. 29:13–14). When a man is willing to set aside the legitimate appetites of the body to concentrate on the work of praying, he is demonstrating that he means business, that he is seeking with all his heart, and will not let God go unless He answers.

This thought of fasting as being an expression of wholeheartedness is clear from Joel's call to the nation:

> "Yet even now," says the Lord, "return to me with all your heart, with fasting." (Joel 2:12)

Says Andrew Murray:

> Fasting helps to express, to deepen, and to confirm the resolution that we are ready to sacrifice anything, to sacrifice ourselves to attain what we seek for the kingdom of God.[1]

Closely related to this is the idea of fasting as giving power to a demand, of bringing pressure to bear in support of one's request. There was an ancient Irish custom of "fasting against or upon a person," which meant "to sit without food or drink at the door of a debtor, or any person who refused to satisfy a lawful demand."[2] Outside the spiritual realm this is seen in fasts that have been undertaken by politicians, prisoners, or others, to bring pressure to bear on authorities and to obtain desired ends.

Without doubt this is an important aspect of the fasting prayer. Of course, we must not think of fasting as a hunger strike designed to force God's hand and get our own way! Prayer, however, is much more complex than simply asking a loving father to supply his child's need. Prayer is warfare! Prayer is wrestling! There are opposing forces. There are spiritual crosscurrents. When we plead our case in the court of heaven, when we cry to the Judge of all the earth, "Vindicate me against my adversary" (Luke 18:3), that adversary is also represented in court (Job 1:6, 2:1 ; Zech. 3:1). It is not enough that the Judge is willing; there is the opposition that must first be overcome.

This is a realm of deep mystery. Scripture states the facts but does not explain them. Importunity is needful in the spiritual realm. Often pressure has to be maintained before the breakthrough comes in the heavenly warfare. There are situations that call for "men of violence" who take the kingdom by force (Matt. 11:12). And all this is no reflection on the willingness of the Most High to fulfill the desires of those who fear Him. Fasting is calculated to bring a note of urgency and importunity into our praying, and to give force to our pleading in the court of heaven.

The man who prays with fasting is giving heaven notice that he is truly in earnest; that he will not give up nor let God go without the blessing; that he does not intend to take "no" for an answer. Not only so, but he is expressing his earnestness in a divinely appointed way. He is using a means that God has chosen to make his voice to be heard on high.

Fasting was sometimes the climax of earnest and prolonged supplication. When the heavens remained as brass despite earnest and persistent prayer, men were sometimes driven in their desperation to fasting as the only solution.

The Benjamites committed a terrible crime, and God told the other tribes to go up against them. They did, and were twice heavily defeated, though they prayed and wept before the Lord. The third time they fasted as well as wept before the Lord, and God gave them overwhelming victory (Judg. 20). What power with God to turn the tide has prayer accompanied by fasting!

Again and again the Israelites fasted in times of national emergency, and what appeared to be certain disaster was averted. And are there no occasions today when death or danger threaten us, that we so seldom employ this means of grace? When Ezra was carrying a large consignment of gold and silver to the temple in Jerusalem along a route infested with bandits, he records, "I proclaimed a fast . . . that we might humble ourselves before our God, to seek from him a straight way for ourselves, our children, and all our goods" (Ezra 8:21, 23, 31). How wonderfully God answered! Do we never face crucial situations calling for divine guidance or protection, that require us to do as Ezra did?

Daniel sought God with fasting for the fulfillment of the promise of the restoration of Jerusalem (Jer. 29:10–13) and received through the angel Gabriel a wonderful unfolding of God's plan for Israel (Dan. 9). If we have sought God in vain for the fulfillment of some promise, it could be that He is waiting for us to humble ourselves and seek Him as Daniel did.

Saul of Tarsus, following his conversion on the road to Damascus, and still blinded by the glory of that light, had been fasting for three days without food or water. His heart was being prepared for further blessing God had for him. Then a disciple called Ananias was sent to lay hands on him that his sight might be restored, and that he might be filled with the Holy Spirit (Acts 9:10–18). Is it some healing touch that we have looked for in vain, despite the assurance of His promise? Or are we still seeking the filling with the Spirit and wondering why our prayers are not heard? We think we are waiting for heaven, but heaven is waiting for us. When heaven can point out the fasting suppliant, and declare, "Behold, he is praying," the answer will surely be at the doors.

In giving us the privilege of fasting as well as praying, God has added a powerful weapon to our spiritual armory. In her folly and ignorance, the church has largely looked upon it as obsolete. She has thrown it down in some dark corner to rust, and there it has lain forgotten for centuries. An hour of impending crisis for the church and the world demands its recovery!

1. Andrew Murray, *With Christ in the School of Prayer*. Fleming H. Revell Co.
2. *The Shorter Oxford Dictionary*. Oxford University Press.

11

To Change God's Mind

*The people of Nineveh believed God; they proclaimed a fast.
. . . When God saw what they did . . . God repented of the
evil which he had said he would do to them.* Jonah 3:5, 10

The power to prevail with God was never more clearly
demonstrated in Bible times than when a pronounce-
ment of divine judgment was averted or deferred through
prayer and fasting. "Yet forty days, and Nineveh shall
be overthrown!" cried the Hebrew prophet. The king of
Nineveh proclaimed an absolute fast for man and beast,
while the people cried mightily to God and turned from
their evil way. "Who knows," ran the royal proclamation,
"God may yet repent and turn from his fierce anger, so that
we perish not." Nor were they disappointed in this hope,
for "God repented of the evil which he had said he would
do to them; and he did not do it."

The Ninevites' repentance, expressed in prayer and
fasting, moved God to change the decree of judgment He
had pronounced against them. This action on the part of
God presents us with a theological poser. God is revealed as
omniscient, as One who sees the end from the beginning.
His foreknowledge is complete and infallible. His character
and counsels are immutable. "I the Lord do not change"

(Mal. 3:6). All Scripture affirms that these are the attributes of the Almighty, and our common sense tells us that without them God would not be God.

Why, then, do so many Old Testament Scriptures affirm that "the Lord repented" or changed His mind? God certainly foreknew, when He sent Jonah, that Nineveh would repent and that its destruction would be averted. This was God's purpose in sending him, that He might extend mercy toward this people. Jonah's message of impending judgment was therefore conditional, though this was not clearly revealed to Jonah or declared to the Ninevites.

God has inflexible laws in dealing with men. Sin is visited with judgment, but repentance with mercy. God has declared Himself on this point in the plainest of terms:

> "If at any time I declare concerning a nation or a
> kingdom that I will pluck up and break down and
> destroy it, and if that nation, concerning which I have
> spoken, turns from its evil, *I will repent* of the evil
> that I intended to do to it" (Jer. 18:7–8).

This repentance of God, therefore, does not imply any caprice on His part, but is wholly in keeping with His intentions declared beforehand. Because man repents in respect to sin, God repents in respect to judgment. Strictly speaking, then, it is not God that really changes, but man. Man's change of heart makes it morally possible for God to behave differently toward him, yet acting consistently with His holy character and principles.

Why, then, does Scripture say that God repented, or changed His mind? This is an example of a common figure of speech[1] in the Hebrew Scriptures by which God's person or action is viewed from the human standpoint. We may think of this as the Holy Spirit's use of language which is an accomodation to our finite understanding. So far as

His declared intentions are concerned, we may say that God repented, for these were conditional; but as far as His character and principles are concerned, "God is not man . . . that he should repent" (Num. 23:19).

After the murder of Naboth and Ahab's compulsory acquisition of his vineyard, God sent Elijah to pronounce divine judgment upon him. "When Ahab heard those words, he rent his clothes, and put sackcloth upon his flesh, and fasted." God then declared, "Because he has humbled himself before me, I will not bring evil in his days; but in his son's days" (1 Kings 21:27–29). Judgment was deferred because even such a man as Ahab was prepared to humble his soul with fasting. How great is God's mercy! How great the power of fasting to call it forth!

David had evidently grasped this fact concerning prayer and fasting. Because of his grievous sin in the matter of Uriah, God had said that his baby son, born of Bathsheba, would die. When the child sickened, David knew that if there was anything that could alter the decree of judgment it was prayer and fasting. "David therefore besought God for the child; and David fasted, and went in and lay all night upon the ground." After the death of the baby, David explained:

> "While the child was still alive, I fasted and wept; for
> I said, 'Who knows whether the Lord will be gracious
> to me, that the child may live?'" (2 Sam. 12:16, 22)

Among the nations of the West, we are witnessing a rising tide of godlessness and lawlessness, similar to that which culminated in the wiping out of civilization by the flood. The sins which brought fire and brimstone from heaven upon Sodom and Gomorrah are fast becoming socially acceptable. Those who should be preachers of righteousness and upholders of the law of God speak out in defence of "the new morality." Surely the writing is upon the wall. The overtones of coming judgment are clear enough to those who have ears to hear.

Even if heaven has issued the decree and the wheels are already in motion, there is still a mighty weapon to which we may have recourse.

> "Yet even now," says the Lord, "return to me with your heart, with fasting, with weeping, and with mourning; and rend your hearts and not your garments."

And then the prophet adds, as though by way of explanation:

> "Who knows whether he will not turn and repent, and leave a blessing behind him?" (Joel 2:12–14)

It seems clear from the prophetic Scriptures that ultimately judgment must fall upon the Christ-rejecting nations. Even Nineveh was ultimately overthrown. But if God can find those who will stand in the gap, even in this eleventh hour, and humble themselves with prayer and fasting, there may yet be a lengthening of our tranquility. God may yet turn and repent and leave a blessing behind Him, giving us mercy instead of wrath, and revival instead of judgment. Such a deferring of the evil day could mean the salvation of multitudes, but there is no time to be lost.

1. An anthropopathism, which ascribes to God the feelings of man.

12

To Free the Captives

Is not this the fast that I choose: to loose the bonds of wickedness, to undo the thongs of the yoke, to let the oppressed go free, and to break every yoke? Isaiah 58:6

"In the day of your fast you . . . oppress all your workers" (or "exact all your labours," KJV), God declared through Isaiah (58:3). Years later Christ said of the scribes and Pharisees, "They bind heavy burdens, hard to bear, and lay them on men's shoulders" (Matt. 23:4), and this despite the fact that they were punctilious in the observance of their weekly fasts.

In this wonderful verse which is the theme of our chapter, God reveals through Isaiah that the nature of the fast that He has chosen is the very opposite. It is not to bring men into bondage but to loose them from it; not to be an instrument of oppression but of liberation. If this word does not have a literal application for us who live in lands where there is little to be seen of the grosser forms of social injustice, it surely has an application in the spiritual realm. Men are bound, not with steel chains or iron fetters, but with the invisible shackles of evil. They fight oppression which is not social but spiritual, even satanic.

In these days when the Spirit of God is moving and the

power of God is being released, evil forces that have lain dormant in human breasts for years are being compelled to throw off their camouflage and manifest themselves for what they are. The discerning eye can recognize that many whom we meet in the path of life are oppressed by the devil, vexed by demons, bound by forces that they do not understand and from which they cannot break free. In many cases they loathe themselves for their actions, weep with sheer frustration at their own impotence to break the chains, and pray as best they know how for deliverance.

An increasingly large proportion of the younger generation are hopelessly bound by nicotine, alcohol, drugs, sex desire and the gambling fever. Others are deceived and entangled by satanically inspired cults and societies, and by varous forms of black magic, witchcraft and spiritism. Worse still, there are Christians bound by fear, resentment, jealousy and uncleanness, who know full well that they are in themselves a complete contradiction to the liberating gospel they profess—but how to get free? They try hard to pray, to believe, to claim, yet still they are bound.

"Are you suggesting," someone may say, "that the gospel we preach is not enough for the needs of such?" The gospel is indeed enough, but not necessarily "the gospel we preach"; for more often than not we preach a deficient gospel. Forgiveness through the death of Christ, though vital, is not the whole gospel. Often a man in the grip of Satan is incapable of responding to this message. Or if he does respond, he may have his sins forgiven without his shackles being loosed. He is saved without being delivered.

Simon of Samaria wished to procure with money the power to lay hands on people for the impartation of the Holy Spirit (Acts 8:9–24). Just because Simon's case presents difficulties, we should not try to escape from them by the simple device of asserting that he was never truly born again. The facts are all against this, and it obscures the lesson that the incident is designed to teach. The Holy Spirit tells us that he "believed," was "baptized," and "continued with Philip" (Acts 8:13). Here are the same credentials of conversion—faith, baptism and continuance—which marked those first converts on the day of Pentecost (Acts 2:41–42).

When Peter told Simon, "You have neither part nor lot in this matter," he was not referring to his salvation, nor even to the reception of the gift of the Holy Spirit, but to the power to lay hands on believers for the impartation of the Holy Spirit. It was "in this matter" of the gift he desired, the motive for desiring it, and the means by which he sought to acquire it, that his heart was not right before God. Peter did not exhort him to repent of his sins in general, but "of this wickedness of yours."

How did Simon come to be in this "bond of iniquity"? Before his conversion he had a mania for greatness, and through black magic had leagued himself with the powers of darkness to accomplish his ends. No man who has dabbled in spiritism, witchcraft, clairvoyance, palmistry, fortune-telling, and such like, can hope to extricate himself easily from the clutches of Satan. Thus, with Simon there was this "carry-over" from his past life from which he needed to be loosed. How many professing Christians today are like him?

Forgiveness was only one facet of Christ's message. Here, in His own words, were His terms of reference: "He has anointed me to preach good news to the poor. He has sent me to proclaim release to the captives and recovering of sight to the blind, to set at liberty those who are oppressed" (Luke 4:18). Those words were uttered at the commencement of His ministry. After it was over, Peter described to the Roman centurion "how God anointed Jesus of Nazareth with the Holy Spirit and with power; how he went about doing good and healing all that were oppressed by the devil" (Acts 10:38).

When our Lord came face to face with a demon-possessed man longing for deliverance, He did not say, "Your sins be forgiven you." He cast out the demons with a word. When He met a woman in the synagogue who had been bound by Satan for eighteen years and could not straighten her body, He did not say, "Your faith has saved you, go in peace." He laid His hands on her and said, "Woman, you are freed from your infirmity" (Luke 13:12). Today we send the man to the psychiatrist and the woman to the physiotherapist! When the root of their trouble is satanic, how can they be cured by the treatment of mental or physical symptoms?

Christ commissioned His disciples not only to preach the good news, but to heal the sick and to cast out demons (Luke 9:1–2). The seventy reported, "Lord, even the demons are subject to us in your name!" (Luke 10:17). In this highly educated and sophisticated age, we have discarded such old-fashioned notions. In worldly society the devil has been laughed out of court. Among professing Christians demon possession is looked upon as peculiar to Bible times or primitive societies or, at most, extremely rare in our modern society. The devil rubs his hands with glee at our blindness.

How great is the need today for the gift of discerning these spirits, and for the faith and authority to cast them out. Undoubtedly many today languishing in mental institutions need, not drugs or electro-shock treatment, but deliverance in the all-prevailing Name. Many in our churches, cruelly oppressed and tormented by the devil, need to be ministered to by those who know how to set the captives free. Many outside the churches, in the highways and byways of life, driven by the devil, are waiting for those who will come to them with a message and ministry of deliverance.

What of the many today who have fallen among thieves? Are we to leave them in the gutter to welter in their blood? Are we simply to pass them by on the other side? It is certain we need to seek and obtain the heavenly anointing for such a ministry. The servant is not greater than his Master, that he can afford to be without his Master's equipping. We need to be equipped with the gifts of the Holy Spirit to discern and deliver. But this is not all. Fasting is a powerful auxiliary weapon, appointed by God, to break the enemy's hold.

"Is not this the fast that I choose," says the Lord: "to loose the bonds . . . to undo the thongs . . . to let the oppressed go free, and to break every yoke?" The primary reference is, of course, to literal slavery. But for us there is a spiritual application, and we must recognize the vital part that fasting has to play in this ministry of deliverance. This is warfare in the realm of "principalities and powers." Satan is a stubborn foe, and will not relinquish his grasp on the spirits and souls, minds and bodies of men unless compelled to do so. Fasting seems to provide that compelling.

In setting free one who is in Satan's power, a "softening-up" process by prayer is often necessary. A fast undertaken at God's direction will strengthen the intercessor to maintain pressure until the Enemy is compelled to loosen his grasp on the captive. Then fasting will also give authority, when God's moment comes, to speak the commanding word that effects the release. This is one of the open secrets behind a ministry of deliverance from the power of Satan, as we shall now illustrate.

13

They Fasted to Deliver

Can the prey be taken from the mighty, or the captives of a tyrant be rescued? Surely, thus says the Lord: Even the captives of the mighty shall be taken, and the prey of the tyrant be rescued, for I will contend with those who contend with you. Isaiah 49:24–25

Pastor Hsi was surely one of the greatest saints that the land of China has produced. Dr. D.M. Lloyd-Jones, in the Foreword to the one-volume edition of his life, says:

> He was truly a man of God in the real sense of the word. His simple childlike faith, which yet was strong and unshakeable, was astonishing. He took the New Testament as it was and put it into practice without any hesitations or reservations.[1]

Delivered at the time of his conversion from the awful tyranny of opium smoking, God used this man in a ministry which brought deliverance to hundreds of his fellow countrymen from opium and demon possession. Many were healed through the laying on of hands. The hearts of multitudes were thus opened to the gospel, and churches sprang up throughout the region. From the time of his conversion, he took the name of *Sheng-mo*, meaning "conqueror of demons," as if by some strange intuition he knew the work that God had raised him up to do.

Within a few months of his own deliverance came the first great test. His wife, who had given evidence of being influenced by his new-found faith, became demon possessed. She suffered from deep depression and mental torment, and when the time came for daily worship, she was seized with "paroxysms of ungovernable rage." The villagers to a man believed that her possession by evil spirits was a judgment upon Hsi for his sin against the gods. "A famous conqueror of demons!" they cried. "Let us see what his faith can do now!"

Hsi had already learned the power of prayer coupled with fasting in the conflict with Satan:

> He called for a fast of three days and nights in his household, and gave himself to prayer. Weak in body, but strong in faith, he laid hold on the promises of God, and claimed complete deliverance. Then without hesitation he went to his distressed wife, and laying his hands upon her, in the name of Jesus commanded the evil spirits to depart and torment her no more.

Mrs. Hsi was delivered instantly and permanently, and forthwith declared herself a Christian. She became his able and devoted partner in the work of God.

Thus began a ministry which has been rightly described as "apostolic." It was characterized by tremendous conflict with the powers of darkness. Great was the power of Satan let loose against him, but greater was the power of God with him to save, deliver and heal. Whatever the crisis that arose—the need of guidance in some important decision, wisdom in handling difficult people or difficult situations, the deliverance of opium addicts or those possessed by demons, the withstanding of persecution or opposition—Hsi had only one remedy. He gave himself to prayer and fasting. What mighty victories and deliverances God wrought for him and through him! While Hsi was still a Confucian scholar and bound hopelessly by the opium habit, God raised up a deliverer in Germany, another "apostolic man" who was similarly used to set many free from evil spirits. Andrew Murray writes of this minister thus:

> At the time when Blumhardt was passing through his terrible conflict with evil spirits in those possessed, and seeking to cast them out by prayer, he often wondered what it was that hindered the answer. One day a friend, to whom he had spoken of his trouble, directed his attention to our Lord's words about fasting. Blumhardt resolved to give himself to fasting, sometimes for more than thirty hours.

The effect of this divinely appointed exercise is told in his own words:

> Inasmuch as the fasting is before God, a practical proof that the thing we ask is to us a matter of true and pressing interest, and inasmuch as in a high degree it strengthens the intensity and power of prayer, and becomes the unceasing practical expression of a prayer without words, I could believe that it would not be without efficacy. I tried it, without telling anyone, and in truth the later conflict was extraordinarily lightened by it. I could speak with much greater restfulness and decision. I did not require to be so long present with the sick one; and I felt that I could influence without being present.[2]

Thus, the ministry of the German pastor grew in power and effectiveness as he fasted to deliver.

Are there those today being used of God in such a ministry? Yes indeed, an increasing number. A woman of prayer in the north of England and known personally to the writer, records the following:

> I received a letter from a lady whom I did not know, telling me about her daughter who was ill. I invited her to my home, and she recounted how this daughter, now thirty-seven, had made a profession of faith when quite young and had been baptized at fourteen. She took up nursing and went quite wrong. She had a baby, and this tragedy seemed to restore her to the Lord for a time. Then she turned away again saying, "God has done nothing for me; I will see what the devil will do."
>
> She was in a mental hospital, and when her parents visited her she threw grapes at them. She would call her father "Hitler," and her mother "Queen Mary." Then she would lie back on the pillow and say, "Evil spirits! Evil spirits!"
>
> My heart went out to the weeping mother, and I promised to fast and pray for her daughter. On the third day of my fast I felt an urge to cast out the demon from this girl in the name of the Lord Jesus Christ. I received a letter from the mother telling me that my prayers had been answered. Her daughter had been found unconscious on the bathroom floor. When she came round she was healed, although very weak, and was soon after sent home.

There are many such needy cases around us. Are we afraid to face them because we know our impotence and fear the power of the devil? Most of us are honest enough to admit that faced with such cases we would not know what to do. We would prefer to call in the psychiatrist rather than tackle a problem for which we know ourselves to be ill-equipped. At least our escapism avoids the embarrassment and humiliation of failure, of having to inquire of the Lord, "Why could not we cast it out?" But are we really satisfied with this situation? Or what is even more pertinent, is He satisfied?

The Lord surely wants us to know His own deep compassion for these tormented souls. He has given us the authority to deliver them. "In my name they will cast out demons" (Mark 16:17). Do we care enough to fast and pray for their deliverance?

It is true that deliverance is seldom possible unless those possessed or bound are wholly desirous of it, and ready by repentance and confession of any sin which has opened the door to Satan to deprive him of any rights within them. Especially is this true in the case of professed believers. But so often there is this deep desire on the part of those afflicted, but no one to whom they can turn who will use the God-given authority, pay the price if need be in prayer and fasting and command the deliverance.

God give us the vision and the faith in this hour of need.

1. Mrs. Howard Taylor, *Pastor Hsi, Confucian Scholar and Christian*. CIM (now OMF).
2. Andrew Murray, *With Christ in the School of Prayer*. Fleming H. Revel! Co.

14

For Revelation

I, Daniel . . . turned my face to the Lord God, seeking him by prayer and supplications with fasting. . . . Gabriel . . . said to me, O Daniel, I have now come out to give you wisdom and understanding. Daniel 9:2–3, 21–22

Though it is often assumed that visions, revelations and inspired dreams passed away with Bible times, Scripture never asserted that this would be the case, and church history supplies plenty of evidence to the contrary. Such means may not be the normal ones by which God imparts His truth or reveals His will, but neither were they in Bible days. The fact remains that God may now, as much as He did then, speak to men in unusual ways.

In times of revival, the church has witnessed in the outpouring of the Spirit a fulfillment, however partial, of the Joel prophecy:

"Your sons and your daughters shall prophesy, and your young men shall see visions and your old men shall dream dreams" (Acts 2:17, citing Joel 2:28).

A new breathing of the Spirit is being felt throughout the earth. God is again demonstrating His readiness to manifest His presence and communicate His mind in the very ways that Joel predicted. Perhaps He has always been ready, but we have been unprepared.

Is there not here the danger of deception and delusion and even fanaticism? Yes, but that danger has always been present, and it is no greater now than in Bible times when God manifestly spoke in such ways. As God was prepared to "take the risk" then, why should He not do the same again? The devil was busy in Jeremiah's day counterfeiting the true work of the Spirit, for he speaks of those who utter "a lying vision, worthless divination, and the deceit of their own minds" (Jer. 14:14; see also Ezek. 13:6–7).

The fact that there is forged currency being passed into circulation only proves the existence of the genuine. Satan does not waste his time counterfeiting what no longer exists. For every false prophet like Zedekiah, God has His Micaiah (1 Kings 22). For every Hananiah He has His Jeremiah (Jer. 28). To turn our backs on the real because of fear of the counterfeit (an attitude all too prevalent among evangelical believers today) is to set ourselves up as being wiser than the Almighty, and thereby playing into the hands of the devil. Fear is one of his most effective weapons against the true work of the Spirit.

Having said all this, we still do well to proceed with caution. We cannot afford to ignore the warnings of Scripture. Let us believe in these things because the Word teaches them, but let us always test them by the Word. From time to time, John Wesley saw the supernatural at work in his ministry and acknowledged it as of God. His warning is therefore all the more timely and acceptable:

> Do not ascribe to God what is not of God. Do not easily suppose dreams, voices, impressions, visions, revelations to be from God without sufficient evidence. They may be purely natural: they may be

diabolical. Therefore remember the caution of the apostle, "Beloved, believe not every spirit but try the spirits whether they be of God." Try all things by the written Word and let all bow down before it.

Without doubt there is a very close connection between the practice of fasting and the receiving of spiritual revelation. Many non-Christian religions such as Buddhism, Hinduism, Confucianism and Islam practice fasting because they know its power to detach one's mind from the world of sense, and to sharpen one's sensibility to the world of spirit. The abstaining from foods is still an important tenet of Spiritism, as it was in Paul's day (1 Tim. 4:1–3).

In the first chapter of Daniel we are introduced to four young Hebrews who refused to defile themselves with the king's rich food and with the wine which he drank, as these would have been first offered to the heathen deities. Instead, they preferred "vegetables to eat and water to drink." The result was that "God gave them learning and skill in all visions and dreams" (Dan. 1:12,17). They proved to be "ten times better than all the magicians and enchanters that were in all his kingdom." So Daniel, trained from youth to a life of discipline in which fasting played a significant part (Dan. 9:2–3; 10:1–3), became one of the greatest Old Testament seers of visions and dreams.

The New Testament illustrates the same point. It was when Peter "became hungry and desired something to eat" (Acts 10:10) that God gave him the vision that led to the opening of the door of faith to the Gentiles. Having told us that he was "in fastings often" (2 Cor. 11:27, KJV), Paul proceeds to speak in the next chapter of his "visions and revelations of the Lord." The angelic message given to Paul at the height of the Mediterranean storm came after a long period of abstinence (Acts 27:21–24). Certainly the prisoner

of Diocletian in the solitude of Patmos would not have
been living on the fat of the land when he became "in the
Spirit on the Lord's day," and was given the final revelation
of Jesus Christ.

We have not found anything in Scripture to suggest that
we are to *seek* visions, dreams or supernatural revelations, but
the point we are making is that those who give themselves
to seeking God with fasting may find God rewarding them
with such manifestations of His presence. But these do not
constitute the only, or even the most important, aspect of
revelation.

Constantly we are needing revelation concerning the
will of God for our lives. We face situations that call for
divine wisdom and understanding. Pastor Hsi was faced
with a serious crisis in the early days of the opium refuge
work when the supply of foreign medicines failed. These
were vital for the treatment of the patients. In this desperate
situation the thought came to him that maybe God would
use his knowledge of native drugs to compound a medicine
to take the place of the foreign supply. He sought the Lord
with prayer and fasting to show him the proper ingredients.
Mrs. Howard Taylor then records the sequel:

> Very simply it all came to him just how those pills
> were to be made. The drugs were at hand in his
> store and, still fasting, he took the prescription,
> compounded the medicine and hastened back to
> the Refuge. It proved an entire success and entirely
> changed the aspect of the opium refuge work.[1]

Why is it that we do not apply this age-old prescription
of prayer and fasting to meet our desperate situations?

Finally, there is the question of revelation upon the
written Word. We all tend to be bound by traditional
viewpoints. There is urgent need for fresh light to break

out from God's holy Word on such controversial subjects as the church, its nature and function; the work of the Holy Spirit in the life of the believer; the prophetic scriptures and God's future program.

We may read and study, discuss and argue, champion this viewpoint or that, but the need of these challenging days is for that "spirit of wisdom and revelation" that is still given to those who seek God with prayer and fasting. Daniel did this, and the heavenly messenger came to him saying, "I have now come out to give you wisdom and understanding . . . therefore consider the word and understand the vision" (Dan. 9:22–23). Light is needed, and light will surely be given, all the light that we require for these dark days, if we prize it enough to seek it as he did.

The promise given long ago to those who keep God's chosen fast is still true:

> "Then shall your light rise in the darkness and your gloom be as the noonday. And the Lord will guide you continually, and satisfy your desire with good things, and make your bones strong; and you shall be like a watered garden, like a spring of water, whose waters fail not." (Isa. 58:10–11)

1. Mrs. Howard Taylor, *Pastor Hsi, Confucian Scholar and Christian*. OMF.

15

Fleshpots of Egypt

*Would that we had died by the hand of the Lord in
the land of Egypt, when we sat by the fleshpots and
ate bread to the full.* Exodus 16:3

It is said that the quickest way to a man's heart is through
his stomach. Evidently Satan thought that that was
equally true for a woman, for it was Eve he tempted with
the forbidden fruit. "So when the woman saw that the tree
was good for food . . . she took of its fruit and ate; and she
also gave some to her husband, and he ate" (Gen. 3:6). So
it was, among other things, a temptation to eat that en-
compassed the ruin of the race. The cry of man's stomach
helped to drown the voice of God in the garden of Eden.

Satan found he could make a strong appeal to the human stomach, and in the millenniums that followed, he
has pursued this line with obvious success. Even Noah, a
man who walked with God, fell into the trap. "He planted
a vineyard; and he drank of the wine, and became drunk,
and lay uncovered in his tent" (Gen. 9:20–21).

In his old age we find Isaac, the patriarch, despite what
God had revealed to him, favoring Esau rather than Jacob,
and for no nobler reason than the fact that this elder son
supplied his father's table with the food that he liked (Gen.

25:28). Esau in turn sold his birthright for a single meal, and for this he later forfeited also the blessing of the firstborn (Heb. 12:16–17). To what extent was Esau's carnality to be laid at the door of his aged father, who did not discipline his own appetites? It is a challenging question for Christian parents.

The sad story of God's people in their wilderness wanderings reveals a continuous record of failure along this line. Over the matter of food, they murmured, they wept, they craved, they lusted.

"Would that we had died by the hand of the Lord in the land of Egypt, when we sat by the fleshpots and ate bread to the full" (Exod. 16:3).

"O that we had meat to eat! We remember the fish we ate in Egypt for nothing, the cucumbers, the melons, the leeks, the onions, and the garlic" (Num. 11:4–5).

"Why have you brought us up out of Egypt to die in the wilderness? For there is no food and no water, and we loathe this worthless food [the manna]" (21:5).

God's attitude in all this is brought out vividly by the psalmist:

He gave them what they craved. But before they had sated their craving . . . the anger of God rose against them and he slew the strongest of them, and laid low the picked men of Israel. (Ps. 78:29—31)

He gave them what they asked, but sent a wasting disease among them. (106:15)

This lust for food even reared its head in the sanctuary of God, and brought a curse upon the house of Eli. God asked the aged priest with indignation, "Why then look with greedy eye at my sacrifices and my offerings which I commanded, and honor your sons above me by fattening yourselves upon the choicest parts of every offering of my people Israel?" (1 Sam. 2:29).

Though God has given us our bodies and planted within them certain basic instincts, including the bodily appetites, we are required to keep the physical subservient to the spiritual. The body is ever to be our servant, not our master. That lust for food displayed by Israel in the wilderness is still with us. If, as Paul tells us, God was displeased with His lusting people then, and overthrew them in the wilderness (1 Cor. 10:5), why should we think that He is any more pleased with His lusting people today?

For each believer there is a finely drawn line between the satisfying of the normal desires of the body and satisfying that inner demanding spirit, that bondage to a fleshly craving, which is not removed because we try to camouflage it. When we cannot say "no" to the second helping of the food we like, though we do not need it; when we are forever having "snacks" between regular meals; when we crave special foods that tickle the palate and appeal to our fastidious appetites; when, in a word, food is an everpresent temptation to which we constantly yield—then it is clear we are in bondage.

> "All things are lawful for me," but not all things are helpful. "All things are lawful for me," but I will not be enslaved by anything. "Food is meant for the stomach and the stomach for food"—and God will destroy both one and the other. (1 Cor. 6:12–13)

> For whatever overcomes a man, to that he is enslaved. (2 Pet. 2:19)

Paul had some hard things to say to the undisciplined believers at Corinth where such evils as drunkenness and gluttony were seen in their love feasts, so that it became impossible to observe the Lord's Supper (1 Cor. 11:20–22). He reminded them concerning the history of Israel in the wilderness:

> Now these things are warnings for us, not to desire evil as they did. Do not be idolaters as some of them were; as it is written, "The people sat down to eat and drink." (1 Cor. 10:6–7)

Sitting down to eat and drink—and the Holy Spirit calls it idolatry! We are not suggesting that the God who gives us richly all things to enjoy cannot bless our feasting as well as our fasting. The fact remains that the Holy Spirit is here warning us that our sitting down to eat and drink can be idolatry, just as it can be to the glory of God. There has been too much indiscipline in this realm among professing Christians to allow us to think that we do not need this apostolic injunction.

It is a sobering thought that all the sin and sorrow, sickness and death in the world today stemmed, in the first instance, from tasting the forbidden fruit. But God be praised that in the fullness of time there stepped into the arena another Man, "the last Adam." He met the attack of the same tempter, not in the perfect environment of paradise, but in a desolate wilderness; not well nourished by the bounteous provision of Eden, but with a body weakened by prolonged fasting and gripped by intense hunger:

> And the tempter came and said to him, "If you are the Son of God, command these stones to become loaves of bread." But he answered, "It is written, 'Man shall not live by bread alone, but by every word that proceeds from the mouth of God'" . . . Then the devil left him (Matt. 4:3–11).

Where the first Adam failed, the last Adam triumphed. Through His death and resurrection, He has restored to man the paradise he had lost through sin. John sees at last the tree of life, from which man had been driven by his disobedience, growing on either side of the crystal river in the city of God. He tells us of the eternal blessedness of those who wash their robes and so have right to the tree of life, who enter by the gates into the city (Rev. 22). Man, shut out from the paradise of Eden, is restored at last to the paradise of God, through the obedience of the Man, Christ Jesus.

In the meanwhile we have to live in a body subject to temptation. "Eating and drinking," Christ warned us, would mark the days prior to His return, just as they had marked the days of Noah. He told us to watch lest our hearts be overtaken with surfeiting (indulgence) and drunkenness and the cares of this life, and the day of His return find us unprepared (Matt. 24:37–38; Luke 12:45–46; 21:34). His disciples must say no to self, take up the cross and follow Him. What part does fasting play in the disciplining of our bodies? That is a question we must now consider.

1. Mrs. Howard Taylor, *Pastor Hsi, Confucian Scholar and Christian*. OMF.

16

To Buffet the Body

I pommel my body and subdue it, lest after preaching to others I myself should be disqualified. 1 Corinthians 9:27

There are those who are seemingly oblivious to their bondage to food and to the fact that there is here a leakage of spiritual power. They mistake the lust that enslaves them for a natural and healthy appetite. Others are aware but show no alarm that they are slaves of the stomach. The truth that Christian discipleship involves self-discipline in this realm has evidently not penetrated their conscience. Their desire and capacity for food is a big joke. "I can resist anything but temptation," they say.

Many who have fasted would admit that it was the call of God to abstain that found them out. As Martin Luther, an inveterate faster, quaintly expressed it, "the flesh was wont to grumble dreadfully."

In his biography of Rees Howells to which we have already referred, Norman Grubb records how God first dealt with His servant along this line:

> It was at a time when he had a great burden for a certain convention, which was being disrupted by assaults of the enemy. The Lord called him to a day of prayer and fasting, which was something new to

him. Used, as he was, to a comfortable home and four good meals a day, it came as a shock to realize that it meant no dinner, and he was agitating about it. And would it only happen once? Supposing God asked him to do it every day!

When midday came he was on his knees in his bedroom, but there was no prayer that next hour. "I didn't know such a lust was in me," he said afterwards. "My agitation was the proof of the grip it had on me. If the thing had no power over me, why did I argue about it?"

At one o'clock his mother called him, and he told her he wasn't taking lunch. But she called again, as a mother would, and urged, "It won't take you long to have it." The goodly aroma from downstairs was too much for him, and down he came. But after the meal, when he returned to his room, he couldn't get back into the presence of God. He came face to face with disobedience to the Holy Ghost.

"I felt I was like the man in the garden of Eden. I went up the mountain and walked miles, cursing that old man within me." . . . He didn't take dinner for many days after that, but spent the hour with God. As he said later, "The moment I got victory in it, it wasn't a very big thing to do. . . . It is while you still want a thing that you can't get your mind off it. When you have risen above it, He may give it back to you; but then you are out of it."[1]

Where there is a failure to deal with this lust for food, the life is opened to attack along other lines. The connection between overeating and the stimulating of sex desire is common knowledge. The sin of Sodom, as we have already observed, was linked with "surfeit of food." God said of Israel, "When I fed them to the full, they committed adultery" (Jer. 5:7). Earlier He had warned them through Moses that their possession of the land flowing with milk and honey after the wilderness wanderings would bring new temptations—the temptation to rebel against God, to forsake Him for idols:

> "But Jeshurun waxed fat, and kicked; you waxed fat, you grew thick, you became sleek; then he forsook God who made him, and scoffed at the Rock of his salvation. They stirred him to jealousy with strange gods; with abominable practices they provoked him to anger" (Deut. 32:15–16).

Paul insisted on the importance of disciplining the bodily appetites and not making "provision for the flesh, to gratify its desires" (Rom. 13:14). Referring to the marriage relationship, he calls for periods of abstinence, "lest Satan tempt you through lack of self-control" (1 Cor. 7:5). In the verse at the head of our chapter, borrowing his figure from the gymnasium or training ground, which was an important feature of every Greek city, the apostle reveals something of his own inner discipline:

> Every athlete exercises self-control in all things. . . .
> I pommel my body and subdue it, lest after preaching to others I myself should be disqualified (1 Cor. 9:25–27).

To the mind of the apostle, there was not merely the danger of temptation, if the body was not buffeted, but of loss of power in the great contest of life, just as an athlete who failed to train seriously would be hampered on the day of the race and lose the prize. He therefore made it his business to take what practical steps should be necessary to subdue the appetites and desires of the body, that the spiritual might be kept in the ascendancy. How could he expect to win the wreath of the conqueror while continually conquered by his own insatiable appetites?

In the days of His flesh, our Lord and Savior knew what it was to be hungry and thirsty and weary, but He ever displayed that perfect self-control which is the fruit of the Spirit. Arriving in the heat of the day at Sychar's well, He ministered living water to a sinful woman while His disciples went off in search of food. Returning with their provisions, they urged Him to eat, certain that He must be as famished as they were. Quickly He replied, "I have food to eat of which you do not know." Had someone come in their absence and brought Him something? "My food," He explained, "is to do the will of him who sent me, and to accomplish his work" (John 4:8, 31–34).

What perfect mastery of the physical by the spiritual! But had He not fasted forty days and forty nights? Had He not repulsed the tempter's attack when urged to turn stones into bread? Man is not to live by bread alone, but sometimes he may have to live by the word of God alone. Was not the life of Him who "pleased not himself" one of perpetual self-discipline? Does He not still call us to follow Him in the path of self-denial and cross-bearing? But how is it to be done?

"It is a perfectly simple matter," someone replies. "The fruit of the Spirit is self-control. Let Jesus live His life in you, and this fruit will be the sure result." This, of course, is the truth, but it is not the whole truth, as many have had to learn through the discipline of failure. There are often outward and practical steps God requires us to take before this fruit can be produced.

We are indeed to "put on the Lord Jesus Christ" by faith, but we are also to "make no provision for the flesh, to gratify its desires" (Rom. 13:14). It is essential that "we know that our old self was crucified with him" (Rom. 6:6) nearly two millenniums ago, but the nails of the cross do not absolve us from the need of disciplining the appetite. The New Testament Epistles are careful to emphasize this latter aspect as well as the former: "Shun youthful passions" (2 Tim. 2:22); "renounce . . . worldly passions" (Titus 2:12); "abstain from the passions of the flesh" (1 Pet. 2:11); "lest Satan tempt you through lack of self-control" (1 Cor. 7:5).

This idea of a self-imposed discipline is basic to the whole biblical concept of fasting. We have already noted that the only fast prescribed by the Law was the Day of Atonement. "You shall *afflict* yourselves" (Lev. 23:27), was the way God described it. Thus, in the abortive fasting described in Isaiah 58, Israel asks querulously, "Why have we fasted, and thou seest it not? Why have we humbled ourselves [lit., afflicted ourselves] and thou takest no knowledge?" David also records, "I afflicted myself with fasting" (Ps. 35:13).

The value of fasting as an aid to subduing the body and mastering the appetite has always been recognized. The Church of England Homily (1562) suggests that the first end of fasting is "to chastise the flesh, that it be not too wanton, but tamed and brought in subjection to the spirit."

This principle is well illustrated in the life of the early Wesleyan preacher, William Bramwell:

> He saw the possibility that, after having preached to others, himself might become a castaway. By stated fasting, by constant watchfulness, by habitual temperance in all things, he kept the body in subjection, and thereby increased his spirituality and power.[2]

Writing to a friend in Liverpool in 1809 he said:

> The reason why the Methodists in general do not live in this salvation is, there is too much sleep, too much

meat and drink, too little fasting and self-denial,
too much conversation with the world, too much
preaching and hearing, and too little self-examination
and prayer.

One might easily imagine he was referring to the evangelical church of the latter-twentieth century. Men like
Bramwell are a standing rebuke to our easy, affluent age.
What a need there is for us to watch and pray and fast, if we
are to keep under our bodies, conserve our spiritual power
and win the victor's crown!

1. Norman Grubb, *Rees Howells, Intercessor*. CLC Publications.
2. James Sigston, *William Bramwell*.

17

What about Asceticism?

Why do you submit to regulations, "Do not handle, Do not taste, Do not touch". . . according to human precepts and doctrines? These have indeed an appearance of wisdom in promoting rigor of devotion and self-abasement and severity to the body, but they are of no value in checking the indulgence of the flesh. Colossians 2:20–23

Perhaps we are wondering if all this emphasis upon fasting, disciplining the body and so on, may not lead to an unhealthy asceticism, or even fanaticism. It is this fear that lies behind much of the traditional attitude to fasting in most evangelical circles. It is a reaction to extremism. Most of us are extremists or reactionaries. In leaning over backwards to avoid the excesses of the extremist, the reactionary falls into the opposite error, and becomes an extremist in reverse. It is not easy to strike the happy spiritual balance of Scripture.

What is asceticism? It is derived from a Greek word meaning "practice or training for the attainment of an ideal or goal," and was applied to soldiery, athletics and learning, as well as virtue and piety.[1] This agrees with the New Testament, and in this sense our Lord Himself, the apostles and every disciplined Christian could be called "ascetic."

Asceticism, however, soon developed features that were erroneous and harmful, and this is why the word carries with it the stigma of extremism in the minds of most people. This is apparent even in the dictionary definition of "ascetic" as "pertaining to the exercise of extremely rigorous self-discipline."[2]

We may distinguish three stages which marked the development of the ascetic spirit in the Christian church. First, there was the periodic and controlled abstention from gratifying the legitimate appetites of the body. Where the motive is right and the method scriptural, this can only result in good, and fasting unto God is an obvious example of it.

Then there was the renunciation of all physical comforts and of normal social intercourse, exemplified by the hermit or monk.[3] The final stage was the self-infliction of various forms of bodily torture, such as wearing a hair shirt or a spiked girdle.

The ascetic spirit, including fasting, is not, of course, peculiar to medieval Christianity. It is found in most primitive religions from the Eskimos of Alaska to the Aborigines and Maoris of Australasia.[4] It was especially common in oriental religions, for example, the Fakirs and naked ascetics of Hinduism. In the development of the ascetic spirit, whether in the Christian or the pagan world, we can discern the master mind of Satan seeking to pervert man's religious instincts.

Behind the erroneous practices of medieval asceticism was erroneous doctrine. There was a false view of God as One who takes pleasure in pain, suffering and hardship. Are there not those today who assume that the hard path must of necessity be the will of God? "Master, I knew you to be a hard man" (Matt. 25:24) summarizes the wrong concept many have of their heavenly Father. Jesus reminded the Pharisees that God would have mercy and not sacrifice.

Then it involves a false view by man of himself, that he can by the rigors of self-mortification atone for his sins or acquire merit with God. This led to the doctrine of penance, and the atoning for sin by "satisfactions" and "merits." Here lurks that insidious pride which glories in its own readiness to embrace suffering instead of glorying in the cross. The one "full, perfect, and sufficient sacrifice, oblation, and satisfaction for the sins of the whole world"[5] needs not to be supplemented by any human suffering.

Finally, there is the wrong attitude to the human body, that it is inherently and incorrigibly evil. Thus, it is deemed necessary, in order to secure the purity of the soul, to free it from all dependence on the body by subjecting that body to rigorous self-discipline.[6] Did the body crave sex expression? This must be ruthlessly repressed by a vow of celibacy. Did it crave sleep? This must be strictly curbed, and so the tolling bell in the night watches dragged the monks from their cells for their vigil of prayer. Did the body crave the comforts of life? Let it be subjected to all manner of hardship, even tortured, for its many sins.

In the monastic system which commenced about the end of the third century, we see the outworking of these false views. There was the solitary monk or hermit, and there was the social who lived in a fraternity where ascetic principles were rigorously enforced. In some communities absolute silence was the rule, and the monks slept in their goatskin clothing in a sitting posture, and declined all ablutions.

Fasting was one of the first things to come under the influence of a rigid and demanding asceticism in the early centuries of the Christian era. Formalism was the thin end of the wedge, while a misguided and intemperate zeal was not wanting to drive it home. Neither Christ nor His apostles laid down any rules for fasting. It was a personal matter between the disciple and his Master, in the light of needs and circumstances. With the decline of vital Christianity, increasing emphasis was placed upon the outward rather than the inward. The form of godliness replaced the power, and men tried to be wiser than the All-wise by supplying rules of fasting which they had failed to find in Scripture.

One fast a year, on the Day of Atonement, was all that the Law had prescribed. But by the time of Zechariah, there were at least four a year (Zech. 8:19), and when our Lord came on the scene, the Pharisees were observing two a week. The history of the church shows a similar trend. What was at first a matter of individual conscience became a matter of custom, such as the practice of fasting each Wednesday and Friday; this in turn became a matter of obligation. Manuals of instruction, based on supposed apostolic authority, brought this and many other matters under rule. "The growth of strictness in fasting is especially observable in the 4th century, the age of councils and organization, made possible by the cessation of persecution.[7]

We are now living in a day of selfish ease and comfortable affluence. Wherever God is pleased to move by His Spirit, there is the danger of a sharp reaction to this easygoing spirit which could quickly lead to an unscriptural asceticism. This tendency lies dormant in the human breast and only waits the right conditions—a zeal which is not according to knowledge and a pride of superior devotedness—to burst into flames.

There is nothing essentially vile in the human body, for God created it, even with its desires and appetites. There is nothing evil in a hungry man's desire for a square meal, or a healthy woman's longing for a husband, children and a home of her own. It is not the way of the Spirit to repress these natural instincts, but to control them and keep them within the bounds prescribed by God. We do not need to extinguish the fire in the grate; only to prevent the coals from falling out and setting the place on fire. The physical is not to be ruthlessly suppressed but firmly disciplined and subordinated to the spiritual.

When asceticism becomes a thing of form enforced by man-made rules, it is incapable of dealing effectively with the bodily lusts. Self-control on the other hand is the fruit of the Spirit, springing from divine life within, cultivated by the habit of a disciplined life.

> Why do you submit to regulations, "Do not handle, do not taste, do not touch" . . . according to human precepts and doctrines? These have indeed an appearance of wisdom in promoting rigor of devotion and self-abasement and severity to the body, but they are of no value in checking the indulgence of the flesh.

Wesley declared, "Some have exalted religious fasting beyond all Scripture and reason; and others have utterly disregarded it.[7] In studiously avoiding the one, let us watch against the other. The much more prevalent error of our day is an easy indulgence which permits us to pamper the flesh when we should buffet it; to feast and enjoy ourselves when we ought to fast and to pray.

Note: The influence of early asceticism on the text of the New Testament is suggested by the inclusion of references to fasting in four passages in the King James Version which are now thought to be interpolations. See Appendix I.

1. *The Encyclopaedia Britannica.*

2. *The Oxford English Dictionary*, Oxford University Press.

3. Greek, *asketes*, from the same root as "ascetic."

4. J. Hastings, ed., *Encyclopaedia of Religion and Ethics* (article on fasting).

5. *Book of Common Prayer* (Order of Holy Communion).

6. This opposition of soul and body is called "dualism." Notice how the revisers ably altered Philippians 3:21, "our *vile* body" to "the body of our humiliation."

7. John Wesley, *Sermon 27* (Discourse 7 on the Sermon on the Mount, Matt. 6:16–18).

18

Fasting and the Body

The body is ... for the Lord. ... Your body is a temple of the Holy Spirit. ... So glorify God in your body.
1 Corinthians 6:13–20

In this and the next few chapters, we shall be dealing mainly with the longer fast and its effect upon the body, though there is much here we need to understand even if we never fast for longer than a day.

Anyone called to undertake a prolonged fast must not be surprised if well-meaning relatives greet the discovery with a look of dismay. This is usually followed by many plausible arguments calculated to dissuade the would-be faster from the dire and dreadful consequences of his foolish course! Sometimes this can be a more formidable barrier than the inevitable discouragements that come from within.

Behind a good deal of the opposition to the protracted fast are the common misconceptions that we must keep eating to live; that fasting is starving; that it is dangerous if not positively injurious. These fears are based on ignorance of a few well-proven facts regarding the activity of the human body during the fasting process.

Food is of course necessary for the sustaining of life, but air, water and sleep are much more urgently needed.

The body cannot live more than a few minutes without air, or a few days without water and sleep; but in normal circumstances it can exist quite satisfactorily for several weeks without food.

Just as the camel has been designed to carry a water cistern within its body, enabling it to traverse the burning deserts, so God has equipped the human body with its own "built-in pantry."

A normally healthy and well-nourished body can exist for several weeks without being injured or incapacitated by lack of food. During a prolonged fast the body is living on surplus fat, and at the same time it is acting like an internal incinerator, burning up the waste and decaying tissues of the body. Only when this refining process is complete does it commence to consume its sound living cells, and that is when starvation begins.

How, then, is one to know when this point is reached? We may usually distinguish three phases through which the body passes during a long fast (though they are not always clearly defined but tend to overlap, and the duration of each varies greatly with the individual). The first phase is marked by a craving for food, which may last for a couple of days or longer. Once it passes, though there may continue to be a pleasurable sensation at the thought of food, there is no craving or strong temptation.

The second phase is marked by a feeling of weakness and faintness which may last for two or three days or even much longer. At this point every movement of the body seems to require an effort of the will. In many respects this is the most difficult part of the fast, and some may find it necessary to rest a good deal. The gradual disappearance of this sense of weakness is a signal that the body has eliminated its grosser wastes and poisons.

The third and easiest is the one of growing strength, with little or no concern about food, and only occasional and decreasing spasms of weakness. At this stage the person fasting often feels he could continue his fast indefinitely without any great effort.

The termination of this final phase is marked by the beginning of hunger pangs, showing that the process of elimination has been completed and now the body is beginning to draw on the sound living tissue. The appearance of hunger is thus the warning bell announcing that the body is beginning to starve. In certain cases this may occur as early as the twenty-first day, but very often it is not till the fortieth day, or even long after. From the commencement of the fast till hunger returns is sometimes called the *complete fast*.

We read of our Lord, that "he fasted forty days and forty nights, and *afterward* he was hungry" (Matt. 4:2). It is significant that the Scripture does not record that He hungered *during* the forty-day fast but at the conclusion of it. This is in exact accordance with what we know of the fasting process, and is thus one of the many incidental testimonials to the truth of the inspired record. Our Lord had clearly accomplished a complete fast, all the reserves of the body had been expended, and starvation was setting in. It was at this point He faced the personal encounter with Satan, and the temptation to turn stones into bread.

It is important for us to distinguish between a desire or appetite for food and a hunger for food. It is doubtful whether the average individual reared in our well-fed Western civilization knows much of genuine hunger. The sensation of emptiness or weakness, of gnawing in the pit of the stomach and other symptoms experienced at the outset of a fast are seldom real hunger. They are a craving for food resulting from the long-continued habit of feeding ourselves three times a day without intermission for three hundred and sixty-five days a year.

When the stomach is suddenly denied what it has been in the habit of receiving as its right, it tends to cry out like a spoiled child denied its after-dinner bar of chocolate. Hunger, on the other hand, is a cry from the whole body stemming not from habit but from need. We might say, then, that mere appetite relates to the immediate "want" of the stomach; true hunger to the real need of the body.

It is strange that any who believe in the biblical revelation should ever have thought that a practice so scriptural as fasting, taught and exemplified by Christ Himself, could ever be harmful to the body, provided it is carried out in accordance with Scripture. The fact is that the very reverse is the case. Fasting makes possible a process of physical therapy. It fully releases the body to operate its own natural system of cleansing and healing.

The loss of appetite, so often the first warning of the approach of acute illness, is thus not only a danger signal, but a signpost pointing the way to recovery. It says in effect, "Stop eating and give your body a chance to recover."

The curative power of fasting has been recognized and applied from ancient times. Plutarch, the famous biographer (ca. AD 46–120), said: "Instead of using medicine, fast a day." Of recent years there has been considerable investigation of this branch of natural therapy by qualified men both on the Continent and in the USA as well as in Britain, and quite remarkable results have been achieved in clinics where "the healing fast," as it is sometimes called, is practiced.

Though the spiritual aspects of this subject are of much greater importance, surely the needs of the body—its health and well-being—are matters that should concern us too.

Our physical condition can often influence our spiritual lives more than we realize.

Because the bodies of believers are the temples of the Holy Spirit, as the apostle reminds us, and because they were bought at such a price, we are to glorify God in them. Is God glorified when they are weak or sickly through neglect of the divine laws that govern their well-being? Is God glorified when we become "casualties" in the fight through overworking, over-feeding or undernourishing our bodies, and failing to give them their "sabbath" of rest and relaxation?

In an age of pressure, when the breakdown of mind or body even among professing Christians is becoming all too familiar, the physical value of a fast of God's choosing becomes a matter of some importance. Here is a divine provision for health and healing, for renewal of mind and body, that we must further consider.

19

For Health and Healing

Beloved, I pray that . . . you may be in health. 3 John 2
Your healing shall spring up speedily. Isaiah 58:8

God has no vested interests in sickness and infirmity. We may say that it is His general desire, as it was the apostle's for his friend Gaius, that His people should be in health. Exceptions to this do not negate the general rule. If this were not the case, He would never have equipped the human body with its own wonderful healing powers or His church with a healing ministry.

Included in the many blessed results of God's chosen fast is the promise, "Your healing shall spring up speedily." Is this a natural healing made possible by the fast, or a supernatural healing? We believe the promise embraces both possibilities.

Fasting, as we have already stressed, has a way of detaching us from the world of the material so that our thinking becomes rightly orientated, focused on God and the unseen world of which He is the center. This inevitably results in a release of faith, which is "the assurance of things hoped for, the conviction of things not seen" (Heb. 11:1).

Scripture has recorded some of the mighty things God has wrought down the years for ordinary men and women who dared to believe Him. They have conquered kingdoms, received promises, shut the mouths of lions, quenched raging fire and even witnessed the resurrection of the dead (Heb. 11: 33–35). It is not therefore surprising that, through the quickening of faith which fasting brings, God has often supernaturally fulfilled this promise of healing.

But there is also the natural healing and rejuvenation of the body through fasting, touched upon in the previous chapter. Here is a natural boon of which all who fast for any reasonable length may partake.

When David and his men were searching for the Amalekites who had raided and burned Ziklag, they came across an Egyptian lying in the open field. Slave to one of the Amalekites, he had fallen sick three days before, and his master had abandoned him to die. For three days and nights, he had had neither food nor water. After he had been revived, he was able to tell his story, and even lead David to the band he was seeking (1 Sam. 30:11–15). It would seem that his three-day fast had healed him.

Surely no one will question that in lands where food is in plentiful supply there are vastly more people who are ill through over-indulgence than through undernourishment. The Edwin Smith papyrus, estimated to be 3,700 years old, quotes an ancient Egyptian doctor as saying: "Man eats too much. Thus he lives on only a quarter of what he consumes. The doctors, however, live on the remaining three-quarters."

From an article in *Christianity Today*, we have the following quotation from James Morrison: "There are multitudes of diseases which have their origin in fullness, and might have their end in fasting."[1] Without a doubt there are ills that could be cured, or better still prevented, and a better state of general health enjoyed if fasting coupled with reformed eating habits were practiced. Oblivious to this, man still continues to dig his grave with his knife and fork!

Earlier we spoke of that deep spiritual purifying that should mark the fast of consecration. This activity in the spiritual realm is being at the same time vividly illustrated—often uncomfortably so—in the physical realm. The purging of the soul is reflected in the purging of the body. The deposits of surplus fat, the waste material and the decaying tissues are being digested and eliminated.

Because there is no new intake of food, the body can no longer engage in the work of assimilation; it therefore concentrates on the work of elimination. Though this may be more marked in the initial stages of a prolonged fast when there is a more rapid loss of weight, the process continues throughout.

Dr. Buchinger, a German specialist on the healing fast, uses the illustration of the Alaskan farmer, cut off by the winter snowdrifts, and with fuel supplies running low, who looks around first for spare lumber, broken furniture, old magazines and books. Then he will have to consider what can best be sacrificed for heating purposes. Only when all that can be spared has been burned will useful furniture be put into the stove. He applies his analogy thus:

> The more inferior the material the less compunction there is about burning it in the fire of metabolism. Gradually, however, after deposits of fat, impurities, and degenerated tissue have been consumed, the body substance can no longer be treated so generously. . . . The delicate inner mechanism carries out work of amazing detail, like a surgeon operating without a knife. In this phase dangerous and stubborn deposits are mostly attacked. Only if the hidden corners have

been cleaned out does the organism have to approach valuable remaining areas of flesh to maintain its metabolism while fasting.[2]

At this point, of course, the fast would be broken off. Only one who has personally experienced this process can truly sympathize with David when he said, "I *afflicted* myself with fasting" (Ps. 35:13). But it is no small consolation to realize that the discomforts we may be called upon to endure in the earher stages of the longer fast are effecting a valuable purifying of our bodies, not to mention the spiritual benefits. This should help us in passing through the rough water to the calmer stretch that lies beyond.

The pores of the skin, the mouth, the lungs, the kidneys, the liver and of course the bowels are all involved, so the medical experts tell us, in this physical spring-cleaning. The unpleasant taste in the mouth, coated tongue and bad breath are all part of the process.

There is the familiar "fasting headache," mostly caused by the reaction of the body to the sudden cessation of tea and coffee—a mild "withdrawal" symptom as the body accustoms itself to being without the caffeine drug. Those who do not use these stimulants are not troubled in this way. Headaches, however, may sometimes have other causes. There is also the tendency to sleeplessness, bouts of abdominal discomfort, nausea, dizziness, and of course weakness.

We cannot agree with those who would have us believe that fasting is either easy or pleasant, something which our nature may enjoy. Nor can we see anything in Scripture to suggest that God ever intended it to be; rather the reverse. It is a physical and spiritual medicine, and our usual verdict on such, however well the pharmacist may sugar-coat the pill, is "unpleasant, but good for you."

What of the general physical benefits? This cleansing process usually produces, after a prolonged fast, a brightness of the eye, pure breath, clear skin and a sense of physical well-being. The digestive system should become like new. A Christian worker after only a five-day fast declared, "I feel as though I've got a brand new stomach." A digestive weakness he had had for years had disappeared.

The sense faculties of the body, especially tasting and smelling, tend to be quickened and sharpened, while one's mental powers become remarkably clear and active. Whatever physical benefits come to us as a result of fasting, it must be stressed that, in so far as our original malaise was due to harmful habits of eating or living, there must be reformation in these realms or the benefits will be lost.

Whether we are healthy or not, we need to get the mind of God before undertaking any fast, especially a prolonged one. Further, we need to have our aims and motives clear and make sure that, whatever we may hope to gain in health and healing, the glory of God and the spiritual issues at stake are our major concern.

1. Quoted in an article, *A Plea for Fasting*, by J. H. Blackmore.
2. Otto H. F. Buchinger, *About Fasting—A Royal Road to Healing*. Thorsons Publishers Ltd.

20

How to Begin

Grant us the will to fashion as we feel,
Grant us the strength to labor as we know,
Grant us the purpose, ribbed and edged with steel,
To strike the blow.
(John Drinkwater)

For the reader who is not content with a mere academic interest in this subject, or a theoretical knowledge, but believes that God now wants him to begin to put some of it into operation, we offer some simple counsel. There are pitfalls, both in fasting and in breaking fast, that should be avoided. We are not now dealing with all the practical questions that arise especially with the longer fast. We have tried to anticipate and answer these in Appendix II. For the moment we are concerned to guide and encourage the beginner.

If you have never fasted before do not start off, as did someone the writer once met, with a forty-day fast!—unless you are very, very sure that God has called you to do this. The body grows accustomed to fasting by degrees, and

God does not usually ask us to run before we have begun to walk, or even crawl. Start with a partial fast (see chapter 4), or else fast one day till supper. Next time extend the fast till retiring, breaking it with just a light meal or fruit only.

When you can manage a one-day fast without feeling faint or famished (we do not say without feeling hungry!), you will be ready for any call of God to a longer fast of three, five or seven days. Sometimes there are spiritual, not to mention physical, purposes accomplished by the longer fast that the shorter does not effect. But the longer the fast you envisage, the more certain you need to be that God has called you to it.

Beware of slavish imitation of others and what they have done, however spiritual they may be. Beware of being carried away by carnal enthusiasm. "Keep back thy servant also from presumptuous sins" must be our constant prayer. Remember that asceticism may be as much "of the flesh" as overindulgence; the latter is a sin of the body, the former of the spirit. When the Pharisees fasted, heaven looked the other way.

If the fast is to be for some days, there is the temptation as it approaches to indulge ourselves while we have the opportunity. "The kine," we whisper to ourselves, "were well fed and fattened before the seven years of famine arrived!" Better far to bend our wills in advance to the battle of self-discipline; that will ease the later conflict.

Some advocate having fresh fruit only on the last day before fasting, that is if the fast is to be for a number of days. Dr. Buchinger, who advocates this, suggests that the "fruit day" ensures that the last meal left in the bowel is fruit, which is less putrefactive than other food residues.[1]

It is wise to cease taking tea or coffee a few days before a longer fast and so get over the caffeine withdrawal headache before you start. (It is wiser still not to return to these habit-forming drinks afterward, or at any rate to take them very weak, and in the greatest moderation.) Other than this, the main preparation you need is one of heart and mind.

It is of supreme importance that you approach this spiritual exercise bearing in mind the principles unfolded in the earlier chapters of this book, and the features that are to characterize the fast of God's choosing. It may help to put to yourself the following questions:

1. Am I confident that this desire to fast is God-given? Would He have me undertake a normal or just a partial fast? "*Jesus was led up by the Spirit into the wilderness.*"
2. Are my motives right? Is there any hidden desire to impress others? "*Your Father who sees in secret will reward you.*"
3. What are my spiritual objectives in this fast?
   Personal sanctification or consecration?
   Intercession? What special burdens?
   Divine intervention, guidance, blessing?
   The Spirit's fullness for self or others?
   To loose the captives?
   To stay the divine wrath; bring revival?
   "*I press on toward the goal.*"
4. Do my objectives tend to be self-centered? Is my desire for personal blessing balanced by genuine concern for others? "*Let each of you look not only to his own interests, but also to the interests of others.*"
5. Am I determined above all else to minister to the Lord in this fast? "*They were worshipping the Lord and fasting.*"

You should expect that a season of fasting would prove to be for you, as it was for your Master, a time of conflict with the powers of darkness. Satan will often try to take advantage of your physical condition to launch an attack. Discouragement is one of his weapons. Guard against it by maintaining a spirit of praise.

Read through Ephesians chapter six and avail yourself of the whole armor of God, then you will be invulnerable to Satan's devices. Make use especially of the shield of faith to quench all his flaming darts. In hand-to-hand encounter, use the sword of the Spirit, and tell Satan, "It is written . . ." Declare the victory of your great Captain over every principality and power.

Do not make the mistake of judging the efficacy of your intercessions by what you feel. Often in seasons of prayer and fasting, you will find the going harder instead of easier, and will seem to experience less rather than more liberty. This is often when most is happening. This is wrestling. This is heavenly warfare. Your Captain did not promise you a walk-over but a fight, and gave you the weapons to win. Often you will not see till later the full results, but the promise stands: "Your Father who sees in secret will reward you."

> From strength to strength go on,
> Wrestle, and fight, and pray;
> Tread all the powers of darkness down,
> And win the well-fought day.
>
>   (Charles Wesley)

1. Otto H. E Buchinger, *About Fasting—A Royal Road to Healing*. Thorsons Publishers Ltd.

21

How to Break the Fast

*They gave him bread and he ate, they gave him water to
drink, and they gave him a piece of a cake of figs and two
clusters of raisins. And when he had eaten, his spirit revived;
for he had not eaten bread or drunk water for three days
and three nights.* 1 Samuel 30:11–12

To break a fast of only a day or two's duration presents
no problem. It is most important, however, that we
should understand the rights and wrongs of breaking a longer fast, and so avoid considerable pain and discomfort. This
chapter, therefore, deals with the practical side of breaking
the longer fast.

The Bible reveals little of how people broke their fasts,
possibly because such matters were general knowledge
in Bible times, for fasting was common practice among
peoples of other religions as well as those of the Hebrew and
Christian faiths. However, we are left with the impression
that the practical side of fasting and breaking fast was not
a complicated business. We should therefore try to keep it
as simple and natural as possible so that the emphasis may
be placed on the spiritual.

The art of breaking-fast lies in the method of bringing
the body back to its accustomed strength and the digestive

organs to their normal efficiency as smoothly and as speedily as possible. With the awakening of hunger and the inability of the body at first to cope with normal quantities of food, it is vitally necessary to curb and control one's appetite until the body is ready for full feeding. This is as great a test of self-discipline as anything faced during the early stages of the fast, for then the food craving was diminishing with each new day; now it is increasing.

Because of the difficulty of this time and also because it is nearly always necessary for the individual, once his fast is complete, to return to his normal work as soon as possible, the "breaking-in" period (as it is sometimes called) should not be unduly prolonged. Unless careful dieting for health reasons is required following the fast, there is usually no reason why one should not be able to cope with any kind of food within seven to fourteen days after the longest fasts, and within a week for fasts of up to twenty-one days, although the quantity of intake will be much smaller than before the fast.

We do not get the impression from Scripture of any protracted season of diet following a Bible fast and before normal life was resumed; and there is certainly no evidence that the period of adjustment was equivalent in length to the fast itself. To insist on this, as some do, would inevitably mean that the fast itself has to be unnecessarily curtailed to allow an equivalent period for returnng to normal feeding, as the overall time that can be given up is usually limited.

Dr. Herbert Shelton, who for years has run his own in-sititution for health fasting in America, must be one of the greatest authorities on this subject. Over the past forty-five years, he has supervised thirty thousand fasts ranging from a few days to ninety days, and for persons of all ages. He reckons to have a normally healthy person back to full feeding within one week after any fast of over twenty-one days.[1]

Whether the period of adjustment be shorter or longer, all are agreed that the utmost vigilance is needed. This is due to the fact that two important things have happened to the digestive apparatus during a prolonged fast. Firstly, the stomach has been slowly shrinking, so that by the end of the fast it has nothing like its previous capacity for food, and the smallest quantity of food makes one feel surprisingly full. Secondly, the organs in the body that are usually engaged in assimilating food have taken advantage of their holiday by going into a kind of sleep which becomes deeper and deeper as the fast is prolonged.

Because of these two facts, the utmost care should be exercised as to *how much* you eat, *what* you eat and *how* you eat it. The stomach must be given time to return to normal size, though this may well be smaller than before the fast. The digestive organs also must be gently and progressively caressed into wakefulness and efficient activity. Clearly, the longer the period of hibernation, the longer proportionately we must allow for the waking-up process.

When should a fast be broken? God will sometimes give specific instructions about this at the time He calls us to fast. Often it is determined by our circumstances and commitments. Otherwise, we may expect to receive direction during the course of the fast, as in the case recorded in the following chapter.

Once you know what the will of God is in this matter, beware of the devil's temptation, usually through difficulties and discouragements, of breaking off the fast prematurely. There is one tragic instance in Scripture of a prophet whom God entrusted with an important mission and told to fast until he had returned from it, who was inveigled by the enemy into breaking the fast before he should have done so, with disastrous consequences (1 Kings 13).

One could, if necessary, break a fast on almost any kind of food, but obviously some foods are much more suitable than others. The two determining factors are what the body can best digest and what will most suitably and speedily build it up generally, at any given stage.

Almost all are agreed that a normal fast (i.e., on water only) of some length is best broken with fruit or vegetable juices, if possible freshly squeezed or extracted, rather than canned or bottled. Many affirm that the citrus fruits are the best. This may well be the case in lands where oranges and grapefruits are picked ripe. But where they are imported the fruit is invariably picked unripe, and the juice can often be too acidic for many stomachs. Apple, tomato or grape juice are possible alternatives, or pure citrus juices canned from the sun-ripe fruit.

Start at first with a small quantity, say a half tumbler, diluted if necessary and taken every two or three hours the first day. Increase the quantity gradually, and then you will be ready to take the fruit itself. Milk can be included at this point, especially in the form of yogurt, which may be taken with the fruit and is highly beneficial.

Fresh salads (without dressing), homemade vegetable soups (no fat) and cooked vegetables may then be included in the diet, always starting with a little of everything new and building up gradually.

A little crispbread or toasted whole-meal bread with a scraping of butter may next be eaten with the meals, but cakes, pastries and cookies should be avoided. Go very steady on the starchy foods at this stage. Protein is best introduced first in the form of cheese, eggs or nuts, with fish and meat last of all. Just how quickly you increase your diet in variety and quantity depends on the length of your fast and how you find the body succeeds in coping.

It is of the utmost importance that the food be eaten slowly, and so masticated that it is reduced to liquid before swallowing. At the first sensation of fullness in the stomach you should stop, even if you haven't completed your portion. Discomfort following a meal should be regarded as a signal to ease off and, if necessary, miss the next meal. This is where self-discipline is needed.

It is important to rest as much as possible during this period so as to let the body concentrate on this business of digestion and assimilation. Resist the temptation to become active too soon. In Appendix II a few other practical matters relative to breaking the fast are touched upon.

Finally, remember these golden rules:

Watch your quantities.
Eat slowly and masticate well.
Stop at the first warning sign.
Rest as much as possible.
Don't try to do too much too soon.

We would do well at this time to give thought and prayer to our future diet and eating habits. We will not want to return to the old ways of undisciplined living, such as overeating, eating between meals, or eating the wrong foods—those that appeal to the appetite rather than those that benefit the body. Of course, we may have no say in this. The question is, "What do I do when I have the choice?" In any case there are several matters which we shall need to watch besides what we eat. A few simple recommendations are given in Appendix III.

One cannot afford to relax spiritually, only physically, during this break-fast period. There must be constant vigilance, for "the thief" will still be on the prowl. Beware of talking about your fast, either how long you fasted or of experiences you may have been granted during it, "that your fasting may be in secret," as Christ commanded.

This should be a time of consolation, when you get right through in prayer on matters that God has revealed to you. You may well experience a greater release in intercession than you knew during the fast itself. You should begin now, if not before, to see the fruit of this time set apart for God, with blessings rebounding not only on your own head but also on those for whom you have been interceding.

This should be springtime in your soul, as well as in your body. It is as though your Beloved is saying: "The winter is past, the rain is over and gone. The flowers appear on the earth, the time of singing has come." New faith, new hope, new love for God and men, new resolves to live only and utterly for His glory—all these should now be burning on the altar of your soul, fed by the fire of intercession.

Thus, like your Lord and Master, return from your fasting wilderness "in the power of the Spirit," expecting that the works of God and the graces of Christ will be manifest in you, as they were in Him.

> "Truly, truly, I say to you, he who believes in me will also do the works that I do, and greater works than these will he do, because I go to the Father. Whatever you ask in my name, I will do it, that the Father may be glorified in the Son." (John 14:12–13)

1. Herbert M. Shelton, *Fasting Can Save Your Life*. Natural Hygiene Press, Inc.

22

Diary of a Fast

THE writer is indebted to a personal friend for this diary of a twenty-one day fast. It is understood that these notes are but extracts from his diary, for there is much that is not disclosed, things that concerned only himself and his Lord. What has been recorded is for the glory of God, and for our guidance and encouragement. It was agreed that these notes should be published anonymously.

Many of the major principles we have been considering are here etched in life: the clarity of the guidance given; the provision of material need during this time; the prominence given to the Word; the spirit of praise when things were difficult physically; the deep personal dealing with God; the emphasis on intercession; specific answers to prayer and the physical experiences varying from day to day.

Those who have eyes only for the sensational may be disappointed. Whatever this contributor may have experienced of the supernatural, he has not, with but one or two exceptions, felt led to record. God may give unusual manifestations of His presence in such times, but we are not to seek after these as though they were the essential ingredient. The value of a fast is not to be judged by how much there is of the spectacular or the dramatic, but how much there is of solid lasting gain for the kingdom of God. According to this principle the fast recorded here will surely rank high in the estimate of heaven.

Preparation

April 1

The Lord is speaking to me about a prolonged time of waiting on Him, with fasting. Therefore, I am cutting out the drinking of tea and coffee in preparation. I need from the Lord a clear revelation of His will for the future, a greater knowledge of Himself and the supply of needs for God's work which call for special intercession. Today I was handed a book on prayer and fasting, and thanked the Lord for this confirmation. I need to know His will when to start.

April 2

Read the book on prayer and fasting, and found it most instructive.

April 4

While in prayer today, I asked the Lord when He wished me to start the fast, and the twenty-fourth day of the month was impressed on my heart. He will confirm.

April 5

In prayer today I asked God to confirm the twenty-fourth. After prayer, went for the mail. There was a letter from R—— who wrote saying that the Lord had impressed the twenty-fourth day of the month on his heart and, although he did not understand why, felt he should write to me as it may have some special significance. Hallelujah! That confirms the date.

April 8

In prayer with my wife today, she mentioned a verse which had been given to her by a friend: "Tarry at Ephesus until Pentecost." Looked in my diary, and found that it was forty days from April the twenty-fourth until Whit Monday. The Lord spoke to me today through my reading in Ezekiel 3:24–27: "Then the spirit entered into me, and set me upon my feet, and spake with me, and said unto me, Go, shut thyself within thine house. But thou, O son of man, behold, they shall put bands upon thee, and shall bind thee with them, and thou shalt not go out among them: and I will make thy tongue cleave to the roof of thy mouth, that thou shalt be dumb, and shalt not be to them a reprover: for they are a rebellious house. But when I speak with thee, I will open thy mouth, and thou shalt say unto them, Thus saith the Lord God: He that heareth, let him hear; and he that forbeareth, let him forbear: for they are a rebellious house."

The Spirit witnessed this to me. The waiting time has to be here at home. The remaining scriptures are so relevant to present circumstances.

April 23

The Lord spoke to me today through Daniel 10:12: "For from the first day that thou didst set thine heart to understand, and to chasten thyself before thy God, thy words were heard." [Here follows a list of things which the Lord had done from April 1 in response to prayer.]

First day (April 24)

Read in Chronicles about Solomon determining to build, beginning the building and finishing the work. This is the day of beginning. Got through a lot of work and study and waiting upon the Lord. A—— called with a sack of potatoes, large box of groceries and £25 cash. How wonderfully kind of the Lord to supply this loving provision for the family. Several callers and a number of phone calls. Drank about six cups of warm water. Feeling well. Went to bed at 10:00 p.m.

Second day

Intercession today for many things [listed in diary] and for the country of ____. Many thoughts given from the Word. Had five people call at various times for counsel, etc. Hunger at times. Drank eight glasses of water. Worked for twelve hours and then had time with some who called. Woke in night with some discomfort but on the whole slept well.

Third day

Much time in waiting on the Lord, and intercession and in the Word. Several people called. Much work done.

Feelings of weakness with occasional pangs of hunger. Body feels the cold in an increased way. Drank fair quantities of water, hot and cold.

Fourth day

Much happened today in contact with others which is a fulfillment of what the Lord indicated some time ago. Wonderful how the Lord is sending people in these days and to see Him outworking His plans. Much blessed in going through the Sermon on the Mount. Listed all the instructions Jesus gave for us to obey. Liberty in prayer.

More feeling of physical discomfort and feeling the cold very much. No real hunger pangs. Cooked breakfast for the family without temptation!

Fifth day

In the Word and prayer. Read Dr. Tozer's *Wingspread*, biography of A.B. Simpson, a man who had to walk the path of "no reputation," but God through him founded one of the greatest missionary societies, The Christian and Missionary Alliance.

Most uncomfortable day as yet, with backache and general feeling of weakness and nausea. Must all be part of the internal process of breaking up of toxins, etc. Also found it more difficult to absorb mentally, but the Lord is my strength.

Sixth day

Another day of work, waiting on the Lord and intercession. X telephoned to get right with me on something he had done, because of the fear of man. The Lord bless him—He always does bless the humble. The servant of the Lord must not strive—God outworks His wonderful purposes—we have the key—prayer.

Still discomfort and weakness today, but count it all joy as this is all in the plan.

Seventh day

Although there is liberty in prayer, I know there is a much deeper place in intercession to be reached. In response to prayer I believe the Lord is sending in the amounts for the work. A. called this afternoon and we had two hours' fellowship together with a weeping before the Lord in prayer and intercession.

A general improvement physically. A few periods of weakness and feeling of heaviness. Since commencement of fast have had no headaches. Noticeable loss of weight.

Eighth day

Spent much of the day in matters related to the work, and in prayer. Read the booklet, *What Really Happened at Azusa Street*, the story of the movings of the Holy Spirit at the beginning of the century in America. Five friends called this evening, and we had a wonderful time together in the Lord's presence. Interceded for some in great need, and for the country. The Lord's presence was very, very real. Certain gifts of the Spirit were in operation.

A definite change today physically, and feeling of re-strengthening. Continue daily to drink fair amounts of water. Cannot say there is no desire for food, but there is no craving for it.

Ninth day

Great liberty in worship, and much brokenness as the Holy Spirit gave a glimpse of the sufferings of the Lord. "What are these wounds in thine hands?" He was wounded for my transgressions. How terrible is sin. I want a greater hatred of it.

More alert mentally today, and feeling much stronger, with lapses of weakness.

Tenth day

Deep heart searchings today, and revelation of the deceitfulness of the heart. Praise God for the blood of Christ. Much work done. Several callers. X called, and he was released. God is answering prayer. A—— also called for prayer—the Lord is sending people. Increase in strength. Drinking about five or six glasses of water daily, mostly warm water.

Eleventh day

Another day of intercession for the nation and for the work in other lands. A—— called again today, and we had a precious time in prayer. S—— and I sought the Lord together in the evening with much liberty.

Feeling very much stronger. Body thin, but heart filled with His goodness. Having about eight hours' sleep each night.

Twelfth day

Much is happening in these days in fulfillment of what God has said in Ezekiel and also in God's original call to me some years ago: "They shall fight against thee, but they shall not prevail against thee, for I am with thee to deliver thee, saith the Lord." Grateful when we can lovingly pray for those who speak against us. "We rest on Thee, our Shield and our Defender." A—— called again, and we spent time in prayer together. Read Daniel, and the Lord spoke to me relative to Daniel's fast of twenty-one days. Know I have to spend forty days set apart to seek the Lord; the length of the fast He will show. Willing for all that He reveals.

Physically this has been the best day yet—feeling strong, continuing to drink six or more glasses of water per day.

Thirteenth day

The emphasis is on waiting on the Lord. After Daniel had fasted for three weeks, the revelation came to him of that which should befall the people in the last days. Seeking His will for the furtherance of the work in the country of ____.

The Lord is faithfully meeting every need. Increasing strength, no discomfort. Praise the Lord.

Fourteenth day

Letter received today from the country of ＿＿＿＿. Been praying for this land and here is an answer toward the future. Blessed by reading Andrew Murray's *Waiting on God*.

Physically a good day again. No feeling of weakness. Weighed myself—have lost twenty pounds in fourteen days.

Fifteenth day

Good day's work. Two friends called, and we had a profitable time in prayer and discussion. Wonderful to see the answers to prayers in matters for which we are interceding. Almost daily the Lord sends gifts toward the work of outreach.

Seem to be on an even keel. No weakness, occasional feeling of discomfort but only for very brief periods.

Sixteenth day

Much work and study done today. How precious is the Word of God, and what a blessed teacher the Holy Spirit is! Reading of the ministries of John the Baptist and Elijah. How we need the voices crying in the wilderness today and pointing to the Lamb of God.

Routine today.

Seventeenth day

Day of prayer for the needs of the work. Had a specific financial need. The Lord sent someone this evening with amount to meet the need, praise the Lord. It is no vain thing to wait on the Lord and trust Him. Real concern in prayer for this nation—like Daniel's mourning for a nation. Slight discomfort today and felt a bit lethargic at times, but so much for which to praise Him for His sustaining grace.

This is not an endurance test, but a wonderful experience of the all-sufficiency of our God.

Eighteenth day

Praise the Lord for another day to experience His strength. The Lord sent over £200 for the work. Very much liberty in prayer and intercession.

A good day physically.

Nineteenth day

Continually impressed by Daniel's fast of twenty-one days. The Lord will show. Much blessed in the reading of the Word in Chronicles and Luke's Gospel. X called again today, and we sought the Lord together. So much appreciated this fellowship in these days. He brought me Watchman Nee's *The Normal Christian Church Life*. How we need a new vision of Christ and His church.

Good day. One feels that one could continue fasting for many days if called to do so. No desire for food whatsoever. Continue to drink about six glasses of warm water a day. Who said that water was tasteless?

Twentieth day

Much impressed in reading of the rich man in Luke 12 today, with the lesson of the parable: "So is he that layeth up treasure for himself, and is not rich toward God." "Thou fool"—God help us to be rich toward Him. Further answers to prayer. A—— called again today for prayer fellowship. D—— called and in conversation asked questions on Daniel 10. He knew nothing of my thoughts on this chapter which mentions the twenty-one day fast, but believe the mention of it was from the Lord.

Routine, apart from a very brief time of slight dizziness. Feeling strong.

Twenty-first day

Gracious words from the Lord through First Chronicles 22:11–19. Believe He would have me terminate the fast tomorrow. He knows the program He has arranged for me next month. I—— called today from W——. Good prayer fellowship together.

Breaking the Fast

First day

Rose at 2:00 a.m. to read and pray. Sought the Lord's confirmation about ending the fast. He gave His peace as His confirmation. Returned to bed, and in the morning the Lord gave another confirmation of His will. Busy day—more answers to prayer. Deep intercession with cryings for this nation.

Broke fast by drinking a little apple and orange juice, diluted with water, and also some tomato juice. NO solids.

Second day

Believe the last three weeks have been a preparation for this day. As I waited on the Lord, He gave me a great burden for this nation, also a vision of a great burning mountain, and out of the bowels of this mountain came forth the judgments of God. Cried to God for mercy upon this country, pleading that He would withhold His judgments until revival came. Know the Lord heard. Cannot describe in words what this day has been. He is the God who heareth prayer—a God of mercy.

Drank fruit juices today. Feeling very strong and mentally very alert.

The return to a full and normal diet was gradual. It was many weeks before I was back to normal weight, but physically there was no deterioration, but an improvement in health.

In Retrospect

The purpose of the fast was not so much to receive but to give, in waiting on God in prayer and intercession. The main purpose was to intercede for the country of _____ and for gospel outreach to another nation. Sufficient to know His purposes fulfilled, reward enough to know the joy of His presence and fellowship with the Lord.

One can now see that since those days of prayer and fasting there has been an ever-increasing ministry of deliverance for others, and at times a new authority in the preaching of the Word. New doors to nations were opened for ministry, and there has been an enlargement in prayer and intercession. However, one cannot go on looking back but must live one day at a time, "looking unto Jesus, the author and finisher of our faith." Fasting and prayer was part of the life of our Lord while here on earth, and "he that saith he abideth in Him ought himself also so to walk even as He walked."

23

In the Last Days

I will pour out of my spirit. Joel 2:28
I will build my church. Matthew 16:18
I will come again. John 14:3

To cooperate with God in the outworking of His plan demands an understanding of that plan. There are three realms of truth which, perhaps more than any others, have been storm centers of controversy among earnest Christians: the doctrine of the Spirit, the doctrine of the church and the doctrine of Christ's second advent (with associated events). This is not surprising if, as we believe, these doctrines hold the vital keys to God's world program. Satan cannot afford to see these keys drop into the hands of the church without a fight, for they spell destruction to the kingdom of darkness. The divisive tactics of Satan, however, cannot thwart the purpose of God.

It is deeply significant that in recent years there has been a worldwide resurgence of interest in the ministry of the Holy Spirit, and especially the pouring out of the Spirit in revival power. But this has forced many thinking people to make a fresh appraisal of their doctrine of the church. If we are to have the new wine of the Spirit, what about the new wineskin? In addition, the swiftly moving ecclesiastical situation, dominated by ecumenism, is sending many back to the New Testament to reexamine God's original plan for His church.

What about unfulfilled prophecy and the return of Christ? Widespread interest in this aspect of truth is yet to come. Let us now see how these three vital keys to God's plan are also closely associated with the subject of fasting.

The Outpouring of the Spirit

Many believers in these days are coming into a transforming experience of the power and gifts of the Holy Spirit. Many others, convinced that a widespread visitation of the Spirit in revival power is the only answer to the spiritual need of this hour, are pleading the promise of Joel which Peter quoted on the day of Pentecost:

> "And in the last days it shall be, God declares, that I will pour out my Spirit upon all flesh."

What shall we say about this? Did the events at Pentecost exhaust the Joel prophecy? Obviously not, or there would have been no further outpourings. Is, then, the final fulfillment in some future day when the church is no longer here? Peter said it would happen "in the last days." Are we not now in what Scripture calls "the last days"?

Some would say that the final fulfillment will be upon Jews only. But the promise says "upon all flesh," and Peter surely confirmed this by saying, "The promise is to you and to your children [Jews] and to all that are far off [Gentiles]." Did he not later witness the outpouring upon the Gentiles, and declare, "The Holy Spirit fell on them just as on us at the beginning"? If, then, the former rain included Gentiles, why not the latter rain?

Almost all are agreed that a visitation of the Spirit upon the church is desperately needed. Are we to believe that the promise to Joel has nothing to say to this situation? Are these apparently spontaneous pleadings for the outpouring of the Spirit from all over the world entirely misguided and out of the will of God? What, then, is the answer to the barrenness and impotence of the church if it is not a visitation from on high?

If, however, we believe that this wonderful promise is for us—is in fact God's answer to the present need—it is vital that we fulfill the conditions as well as plead the promise. Three times Joel sounds a clarion call, in view of the imminence of the Day of the Lord, to return to God *with fasting* (1:14; 2:12, 15). Then he seems to see in vision God's response: "Then the Lord became jealous for his land, and had pity on his people" (2:18), granting deliverance and prosperity, followed by the outpouring of the Spirit on all flesh. Have we any right to expect the fulfillment of this wonderful promise without obedience to the conditions? Have we yet prayed "with all our hearts, even with fasting"? Have tears ever been mingled with our prayers? Have the priests, the ministers of the Lord, ever wept between the porch and the altar? The promised outpouring calls for fasting as well as prayer.

The Restoration of the Church

Some five hundred years before Christ, the exiled prophet Daniel observed from the study of Jeremiah's prophecy that the time was at hand when God would bring His people back to Jerusalem (Dan. 9:2; Jer. 29:10). He therefore sought God in prayer with fasting and sackcloth and ashes, that He would fulfill the promise. Confession mingled with his supplication as he prayed that God would cause His face to shine upon His sanctuary which was desolate.

This fasting prayer of Daniel set the wheels in motion that led to one of the most remarkable decrees that a heathen king ever issued. Cyrus made a proclamation to the effect, that God had charged him to build Him a house in Jerusalem, and that those Jews who were so disposed were to go up to Jerusalem to rebuild the house of the Lord (Ezra 1:14). So there came about the first return of the exiles under Zerubbabel to rebuild the temple. Again, prayer and fasting under the good hand of God had changed the course of history. In the later expedition under Ezra, fasting again played its part in the safe arrival of the exiles with their precious consignment for the house of God (8:21–23).

Under the old covenant God had a temple for His people; under the new God has His people for a temple. As we look out today on the church, God's spiritual habitation, what a need for spiritual renewal! If the early Christians were still with us, God might well ask, "Who is left among you that saw this house in its former glory? How do you see it now? Is it not in your sight as nothing?" (Hag. 2:3). The restoration of the church to its former power and glory would involve a transformation no less radical than that which took place in the temple long ago under Zerubbabel and Ezra. Did not God encourage His people with the promise, "The latter splendor of this house shall be greater than the former"? (2:9).

The outpouring of the Spirit is not enough. The new wine must have now, as it had when poured out on the day of Pentecost, a new wineskin. The renewing of the house of God is indispensable. It cost these men of the Old Testament deep intercession with fastings and tears. Would we think to obtain it more cheaply—by consultations and conversations and committees?

The Return of Christ

Neither the outpouring of the Spirit nor the reformation of the church is our goal. It is nothing less than "the prize of the upward call of God in Christ Jesus." The supreme hope of the church lies in the promise of the reappearance of the Lord from heaven. He told His disciples, "I will come again." Clearly this coming was not spiritual but visible and literal, for as the angels informed the apostles, "This Jesus, who was taken up from you into heaven, will come in the same way as you saw him go into heaven" (Acts 1:11).

Here is the grand and glorious consummation of the age, for which all that proceeded it was a necessary preparation. Do we long for His return? Do we share what must be the yearning of His heart for that coming day of vindication and coronation? When He summons us in that day to account for our talents, will we have to confess that the fasting talent was never used, that we hid this precious entrustment in the ground?

Fasting, then, opens the way for the outpouring of the Spirit and the restoration of God's house. Fasting in this age of the absent Bridegroom is in expectation of His return. Soon there will be the midnight cry, "Behold, the bridegroom! Come out to meet him." It will be too late then to fast and to pray. The time is now.

They Fasted

On Sinai's mount, with radiant face,
To intercede for heaven's grace
Upon a stubborn, wayward race,
    He fasted.

Once lifted from the miry clay,
When opposition came his way
This soldier-king would often pray
    With fasting.

A seer, possessed of vision keen,
Who told the troubled king his dream,
Had light on God's prophetic scheme
    Through fasting.

The prophetess in temple court
Beheld the Babe the two had brought;
For Him she long had prayed and sought,
    With fasting.

He came to break the yoke of sin,
But ere His mission could begin
He met the foe and conquered him
    With fasting.
"Set these apart," the Spirit bade.
A spring, that soon vast rivers made,

Broke ope by men who as they prayed
    Were fasting.

"So shall they fast when I am gone";
Was this no word to act upon?
Ask countless saints who fought and won
    With fasting.

When we shall stand on that great day
And give account, what shall we say,
If He should ask us, "Did you pray
    With fasting?"

                     (A.W.)

Appendix I

Doubtful References to Fasting
in the King James Version

There are four verses in the New Testament where the King James Version has a reference to fasting not endorsed by more recent scholarship, and therefore omitted in later translations.

The following versions and translations, given in chronological order, were consulted:

The New Translation by J.N. Darby, 1871
The Revised Version (RV), 1885
The American Standard Version (ASV), 1901
The New Testament in Modern Speech by R.F.
    Weymouth, 1902
The New Translation by James Moffatt, 1913
The Revised Standard Version (RSV), 1952
The New Testament in Modern English by J.B.
    Phillips, 1958
The Amplified New Testament, 1958
The New Testament of the New English Bible
    (NEB), 1961

The words in doubt are in italics.

1. Matthew 17:21: "*Howbeit this kind goeth not out but by prayer and fasting.*"

Only the translations of Darby and Weymouth include this verse. The Amplified New Testament puts it in italics as "not adequately supported by recent scholarship." All the others omit the verse completely. The IVP Commentary says: "Verse 21 is omitted by the more reliable texts. It seems to have been interpolated from Mark 9:29."

2. Mark 9:29: "And he said unto them, This kind can come forth by nothing, but by prayer *and fasting.*"

The words "and fasting" are rejected by all the translations consulted, except for Darby and Moffatt. The Amplified again uses italics. The IVP Commentary, however, while admitting that these two words are not found in Codices Sinaiticus and Vaticanus, does not consider that the evidence against them is conclusive.

It is believed there are internal as well as textual reasons for rejecting these words, and this applies to the parallel verse in Matthew just considered. Fasting, we have sought to show, is not a synonym for self-denial in the New Testament, but means abstinence from food. Either there is a departure from the general rule in this passage, so that our Lord's words only had reference to general self-discipline—in which case we cannot use this verse to establish anything about literal fasting—or, if we take the word literally, His statement conflicts with what we learn elsewhere, that Jesus did not fast once His ministry began nor the disciples while Jesus was with them.

Also, the introduction of the thought of fasting here obscures what we believe was the lesson Jesus was impressing on the disciples through their failure to set free the epileptic.

It was not that a season of prayer and fasting was necessary before this kind of spirit could be cast out—certainly our Lord did not tarry for this—but that had they been living, like Him, *the life of prayer*, they too could have dealt successfully with this case. This of course does not negate the fact that fasting is an invaluable aid to prayer in such cases of deliverance, but this does not appear to be the point Jesus was emphasizing.

3. Acts 10:30: "And Cornelius said, Four days ago I was *fasting* until this hour; *and* at the ninth hour I prayed in my house. . . ."

    "I was keeping the ninth hour of prayer" (RV, RSV) is how this verse is generally rendered, only Darby supporting the inclusion of "fasting." Prof. F. F. Bruce on this passage draws attention to "the pietistic addition of fasting" by an editor who "refuses to leave anything to the reader's imagination" (*The Acts of the Apostles*, the Greek Text with Introduction and Commentary, Tyndale Press, 222).

4. 1 Corinthians 7:5: "Defraud ye not one the other, except it be with consent for a time, that ye may give yourselves to *fasting and* prayer; and come together again. . . ."

    J.B. Phillips, oddly enough, is the only translator to support the inclusion of "fasting" here. Dean Alford points out, under this verse in his Greek Testament, "how such passages as this have been tampered with by the ascetics."

Appendix II

Answers to Practical Questions

1. WHEN FASTING IS INADVISABLE: *Are there some illnesses or conditions that render fasting inadvisable?*

   In cases of serious undernourishment or nervous exhaustion, fasting is not recommended unless for very short periods. It should not be undertaken by diabetic patients, especially if insulin is being taken. Nor is it deemed advisable for expectant mothers. If there is any doubt about fitness to fast, one should seek medical advice.

2. FASTING WHILE WORKING: *Is it practicable to fast while carrying on one's work?*

   That depends on the nature of the work, the length of the fast, and varies to some extent with the individual. There should be no difficulty in undertaking a day's fast, whatever one's occupation. One has known of housewives and mothers who have profited from a fast of three days or longer while running the home, preparing meals, etc., and giving what time they could to prayer. One has known of manual workers who have undertaken longer fasts with no ill effects, but one would not normally recommend it. The ideal is to be as free as possible to seek God at such a time, and to take the necessary rest.

3. FASTING IF UNDERWIEGHT: *Is it unwise to fast if under-
    weight?*

According to Dr. H. Shelton, it is common to find that
underweight people recover their normal healthy weight
following a longer fast. Overfeeding and loss of weight
often go together. One can eat too much and assimilate
too little if the digestive powers are impaired. Fasting will
often remedy this, so that afterward the person may eat less,
assimilate more and the weight return to normal.

4. AVERAGE LOSS OF WEIGHT: *What is the average daily
    weight loss during a fast?*

It varies greatly with the individual. In the first stages
of a longer fast, the graph of one's daily loss is steeper, and
then it starts to level out. Two pounds a day, decreasing to
one, would be quite average, but overweight people may
lose much more. Provided there is sufficient rest, fasting
is the safest, most efficient and certainly the most natural
weight-reducer.

5. FASTING AND THE BOWELS: *Should one use laxatives or
    enemas while fasting?*

The bowel, a twisted tube some twenty-five feet long,
takes on average about twenty-four hours to discharge its
contents. It is quite common to find that after the first few
days, without the stimulation of fresh intakes of food, it
ceases to function. Some recommend Glauber's Salts ($1^1/2$
oz. in $1^1/4$ pints of warm water) on the first day of the fast,
and then periodical enemas. Laxatives are not recommended
once the fast is underway. Dr. Shelton, however, prefers to
let nature handle its own affairs without any forcing by
laxative or enema. He takes the view that if the bowels need

to operate they will; otherwise they may be more benefited by prolonged rest. This seems to be the simpler and more natural course, and what must have been done in Bible times. On a long fast food residue may remain in the bowel for as long as 3 weeks, but while there is no food intake this should not create any problem with constipation.

In breaking a long fast, it may be some days before the bowels start to operate. Again, it is wise to exercise patience and give them time. Once they start they will usually function more regularly and efficiently than before. Some people are helped by taking prunes or figs first thing in the morning, and a daily drink of molasses.

6. FASTING IN WINTER: *Is it advisable to fast in winter?*

While one is fasting, the fire of metabolism is being fed with low-grade fuel and consequently not generating its usual heat. The body therefore tends to feel the cold. Provided one is careful to keep warm, there is no reason for not fasting in winter.

7. DIZZINESS: *Is there any way of preventing dizziness during fasting?*

This is usually a temporary symptom. It is sometimes caused by a sudden change of position, especially sitting up from the lying position. The remedy in that case is to move slowly.

8. SLEEPLESSNESS: *Can one do anything about sleeplessness?*

This is sometimes due to the fact that the mind is overactive. It is wise to avoid any concentrated mental activity before retiring, and resist the temptation to sleep (though not to rest) during the day.

9. FOUL BREATH: *What can be done about bad breath?*

It has been suggested that a small quantity of menthol crystals be procured, and if one is allowed to dissolve on the tongue, it will provide relief.

10. DRINKING WATER: *How much water should one drink during a fast?*

Some recommend drinking as much as possible, on the assumption that this aids the process of elimination by flushing the system. There seems some doubt whether this is the case. Better to let the body determine how much is drunk. Sipping water does help stave off the craving for food and the spasms of weakness. It may be taken hot, cold (but not chilled) or lukewarm. A slice of lemon in the water jug will take away the metallic taste.

11. PRACTICAL MEASURES: *What other practical points should one bear in mind during fasting?*

- A daily shower or bath with warm but not hot water.
- Deep breathing, concentrating on exhaling as fully as possible.
- Regular exercise (not too strenuous), except where there is great weakness.

12. FALSE IMPRESSIONS: *May not a person fasting be subject to impressions and voices which are not from God?*

This is true. Fasting makes one sensitive to the world of spirit, whether divine or satanic. Only if Satan already has avenues in a person's life will he become subject to satanic impressions when he fasts. That these inroads should become evident in this way is often the first step to deliverance for the person concerned. Where there are no such avenues, we have nothing to fear, provided we remain humble before God and are clad in the heavenly armor. God did not design fasting to make us vulnerable to Satan.

Appendix III
Healthy Eating

Dietetics is a vast subject outside the scope of this book. Nevertheless, the practice of fasting tends to exercise our minds on the matter of disciplined eating—both what we eat and how we eat it. "Some people eat to live, and others live to eat." Some eat with their health in view, and others think only of their appetite. Wrong eating is the cause of many ills. To put the thing on the highest plane, we owe it to the God who gave us these bodies to keep them as fit as possible to serve Him.

As to what we eat, we may be in a position where the apostolic injunction applies: "Whatever is set before you, eat, asking no question"! When we are able to choose, while guarding against any tendency to become faddy or cranky over food, we should concentrate on the health-giving foods rather than those which merely please our appetites. This is surely included in the command to eat and drink to the glory of God.

There is a growing tendency for man in his scientific laboratory to think that he can imitate and even improve upon the work of nature. This is particularly true in the food realm. So much that we eat and drink nowadays is canned, processed, refined, preserved, dehydrated, pasteurized or otherwise chemically treated—and supposedly for our safety and good! Dr. Herbert Shelton, speaking from the widest experience in this connection, says:

> The acid test of a food, it seems to me, is its fitness to serve the nutritive needs of the human organism just coming off a prolonged fast. In all my experience with feeding, I have found nothing turned out synthetically by food manufacturers to equal the untouched products of garden, orchard and field. . . . I emphasize the importance of eating fresh, uncooked fruits, and vegetables daily. (From his book on fasting, p. 74.)

Finally, here are a few well-proven rules for healthy eating:

1. Eat to appease your hunger, and then stop. Do not go on to satisfy your appetite.

2. Eat slowly and masticate well. Better leave the meal unfinished than bolt it.

3. Let your mind relax. Intensive concentration, nervous tension, emotional disturbance impair the digestion.

4. Try to develop the habit of drinking between and not during meals.

5. Avoid "snacks" between meals.

6. Avoid a heavy meal late at night. Remember your digestive organs need rest too.

7. Learn what are the natural, health-giving foods, and ensure that they constitute a good proportion of your diet. (Your local bookseller or health food store will advise you of the many publications now available on the subject of food reform.)

8. Avoid tea and coffee (there are plenty of substitutes) or else take them in the greatest moderation. They have no nutritional value, and as stimulants, tend to

be habit-forming. "All things are lawful for me, but I will not be enslaved by anything."

Biblical Index

References to fasting in Scripture, whether full or partial, are given in order, and where the Scripture has been touched upon in this book, the page number is given.

Gen. 24:33	Abraham's servant seeking a bride for Isaac
Exod. 34:28	Moses' first period of forty days on Sinai, 20
Lev. 16:29, 31	On the Day of Atonement
Lev. 23:14	Until the sheaf of the wave offering was offered
Lev. 23:27, 32	On the Day of Atonement, 35, 91
Num. 6:3–4	The law of the Nazirite
Num. 29:7	On the Day of Atonement
Deut. 9:9, 18	Moses' two periods of forty days on Sinai, 20
Judg. 20:26	By Israel after their defeat by Benjamin, 56
1 Sam. 1: 7–8	Hannah's prayer for a child
1 Sam. 7:6	At Mizpah under Samuel, 48
1 Sam. 14:24–30	Saul's curse uttered in battle
1 Sam. 20:34	Jonathan grieved at Saul's hatred of David
1 Sam. 30:11–12	Egyptian servant David found in the field, 106, 115
1 Sam. 31:13	By those that buried Saul and his sons, 48
2 Sam. 1:12	By David and his men at news of Saul's death
2 Sam. 3:35	By David at Abner's death

2 Sam. 11:11	Uriah's self-discipline in time of battle
2 Sam. 12:16–23	By David for the child of Bathsheba, 61
1 Kings 13:8–24	By prophet who cried against altar at Bethel, 118
1 Kings 17:6, 14–16	Elijah's restricted diet at Cherith and Zarephath, 24
1 Kings 19:8	By Elijah on his journey to Horeb, 20
1 Kings 21:4–5	By Ahab after Naboth's refusal
1 Kings 21:9, 12	When Naboth was set on high at Jezebel's instigation
1 Kings 21:27	By Ahab in self-humiliation, 61
1 Chron. 10:12	By those who buried Saul and his sons
2 Chron. 20:3	Proclaimed by Jehoshaphat before battle, 37
Ezra 8:21–23	Proclaimed by Ezra at the river Ahava, 37, 53, 56, 136
Ezra 9:5	Ezra mourning for the faithlessness of the exiles, 19, 48
Ezra 10:6	Ezra mourning for the faithlessness of the exiles, 19
Neh. 1:4	By Nehemiah for the restoration of Jerusalem
Neh. 9:1	By people of Jerusalem, confessing their sins, 49
Esther 4:3	By the Jews following Haman's decree
Esther 4:16	Called by Esther before audience with the king, 19, 28
Esther 9:31	In connection with the feast of Purim
Job 33:19–20	As a result of pain or sickness
Ps. 35:13	David on behalf of others who were sick, 35, 91, 108
Ps. 42:3	When the Psalmist's tears became his food
Ps. 69:10	The cause of David being reproached, 47
Ps. 102:4	The Psalmist forgets food in his affliction
Ps. 107:17,18	As a result of sickness
Ps. 109:24	The cause of David's physical weakness

Isa. 58	The kind of fasting which pleases God, 42, 53, 63, 67, 79
Jer. 14:12	That which is unacceptable to God
Jer. 36:6,9	Baruch reading Jeremiah's scroll on a fast day, 35
Dan. 1:12–16	Daniel and his companions refuse the king's food, 23, 77
Dan. 6:18	Darius when Daniel was in the lions' den, 39
Dan. 9:3	Daniel praying for Jerusalem, 56, 77, 79, 135
Dan. 10:2–3	Daniel's three weeks' partial fast, 24, 77, 135
Joel 1:14	In view of the Day of the Lord, 43, 135
Joel 2:12	When returning to God with all the heart, 54, 62, 135
Joel 2:15	Proclaimed by blowing a trumpet in Zion, 35, 135
Jon. 3:5–9	Proclaimed by the people and king of Nineveh, 37, 59, 60
Zech. 7:3–5	With mourning in the fifth and seventh months, 41, 43
Zech. 8:19	Kept in the fourth, fifth, seventh and tenth months, 35, 96
Matt. 4:2	By our Lord for forty days, 15, 16, 50, 84, 90, 101, 113
Matt. 6:16–18	Not to be practiced as the hypocrites do, 27, 112, 120
Matt. 9:14–15	By John's disciples and the Pharisees, 48
Matt. 9:15	By the guests when the bridegroom has departed, 12, 29–33
Matt. 11:18	The abstemious character of John the Baptist, 25
Matt. 15:32	State of the four thousand before our Lord fed them, 39
Matt. 17:21*	This kind can only come forth by it, 142
Mark 2:18	By John's disciples and the Pharisees
Mark 2:19–20	By the guests when the bridegroom has departed
Mark 8:3	State of the four thousand when our Lord fed them

Mark 9:29*   This kind can only come forth by it, 142

Luke 2:37   By Anna worshipping in the temple, 43

Luke 4:2   By our Lord for forty days, 16, 50

Luke 5:33   By John's disciples and the Pharisees

Luke 5:34–35   By the guests when the bridegroom has departed

Luke 7:33   The abstemious character of John the Baptist, 25

Luke 18:12   By the boastful Pharisee, twice a week, 36, 42

Acts 9:9   Saul of Tarsus after his encounter with Christ, 20, 56

Acts 10:30*   By Cornelius when an angel appeared to him, 143

Acts 13:2–3   By prophets and teachers in Antioch, 28, 32, 41, 44, 50, 113

Acts 14:23   At the appointment of elders in the churches, 50

Acts 23:12–21   By Jews under an oath to kill Paul

Acts 27:9   Allusion to the annual Day of Atonement, 35

Acts 27:21, 33 By those with Paul before the shipwreck, 77

Rom. 14:21   Abstaining for the sake of a weaker brother

1 Cor. 7:5*   In the marriage relationship,16, 89, 91, 143

1 Cor. 8:13   Abstaining for the sake of a weaker brother

2 Cor. 6:5   An ingredient of the apostolic ministry, 16, 39

2 Cor. 11:27   In the list of Paul's sufferings, 16, 39, 77

1 Tim. 4:3   False teachers commanding abstinence, 77

* References to fasting in the King James Version of the New Testament omitted by most later versions (see Appendix I)

This book was produced by CLC Publications. We hope it has been life-changing and has given you a fresh experience of God through the work of the Holy Spirit. CLC Publications is an outreach of CLC Ministries International, a global literature mission with work in over fifty countries. If you would like to know more about us or are interested in opportunities to serve with a faith mission, we invite you to contact us at:

CLC Ministries International
PO Box 1449
Fort Washington, PA 19034

———

Phone: 215-542-1242
E-mail: orders@clcpublications.com
Website: www.clcpublications.com

DO YOU LOVE GOOD CHRISTIAN BOOKS?
Do you have a heart for worldwide missions?

You can receive a FREE subscription to
CLC's newsletter on global literature missions
Order by e-mail at:

clcworld@clcusa.org

Or fill in the coupon below and mail to:

PO Box 1449
Fort Washington, PA 19034

FREE *CLC WORLD* SUBSCRIPTION!

Name: _____

Address:_____

_____

Phone: _____ E-mail:_____

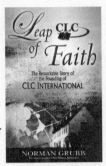

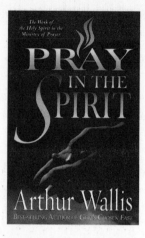

PRAY IN THE SPIRIT

Arthur Wallis

Arthur Wallis sets the pace for a book on prayer, going beyond general principles to show the role of the Holy Spirit in the life of the praying believer. Through a pointed analysis of our struggles in prayer—both our spiritual and practical difficulties—Wallis shows how the Holy Spirit helps us in our weaknesses.

Trade paper ISBN: 978-0-87508-574-6

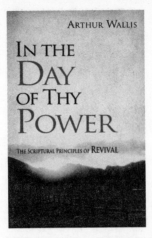

IN THE DAY OF THY POWER

Arthur Wallis

"Oh, that You would rend the heavens! That You would come down!"

Millions have prayed that, and pray it now.

Has it ever happened? Yes,

God has come down; both the Bible and Christian history bear witness to it. *In the Day of Thy Power* is filled with plentiful quotations from eyewitnesses of revival and with inescapable biblical authority for such "times of refreshing . . . from the presence of the Lord." It unfolds the conditions by which God still comes, as in apostolic days, with "mighty signs and wonders, by the power of the Spirit of God."

Trade paper ISBN: 978-1-936143-02-3

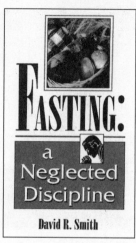

FASTING:
a Neglected Discipline

David R. Smith

Have you ever fasted?

***Has it even occured to you that you
ought to be considering the question of fasting?***

The fact is that the subject of fasting seems to have dropped
right out of our lives, and out of our Christian thinking.

Learn the purpose and benefits of fasting along with the
method.

Trade paper ISBN: 978-0-87508-515-9

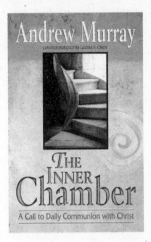

THE INNER CHAMBER

Andrew Murray

Contemporized by Leona F. Choy

"Healthy roots grow healthy branches."

"The neglect of this principle is why so many believers are weak and fruitless," says Andrew Murray.

In his distinctive devotional style, Murray calls us to a daily cultivation of heart communion with Christ, from which we draw the grace to live for Him. This is not a simplistic "how-to" on a daily quiet time, but a challenging exhortation to come alone with our Lord to find strength for each day.

Trade paper ISBN: 978-0-87508-995-9

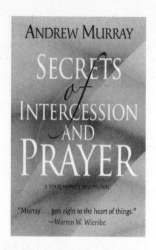

"Murray . . . gets right to the heart of things."
—Warren W. Wiersbe

SECRETS OF INTERCESSION AND PRAYER

Andrew Murray

Have you learned the secrets of the great intercessors of the church?

Do you know how to adore God in prayer?

Do you long to know His abiding presence?

Have you discovered the blessings of praying with others?

Andrew Murray's "Secret Series" booklets have long been classics of devotional literature. Now CLC Publications has collected four of his best into one volume: *The Secret of the Abiding Presence, The Secret of Adoration, The Secret of Intercession* and *The Secret of United Prayer.*

Trade paper ISBN: 978-0-87508-765-8

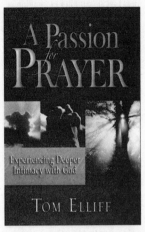

A PASSION FOR PRAYER

Tom Elliff

Of all the disciplines of the Christian life, prayer is perhaps the most neglected. Yet Jesus' brief earthly life was permeated with it. *A Passion for Prayer* seeks to help you develop—or deepen—your communion with God. Drawing on personal experience and God's Word, Pastor Tom Elliff shares principles for daily coming before the throne of grace.

Trade paper ISBN: 978-1-936143-03-0

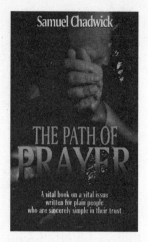

THE PATH OF PRAYER

Samuel Chadwick

What is prayer and what are its functions? This helpful volume is based not on theory but experience, and is simply written so that everyone will be able to apply its principles.

Mass Market ISBN: 978-0-87508-578-4

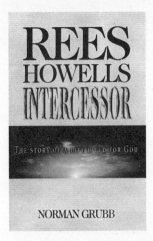

REES HOWELLS INTERCESSOR

Norman Grubb

Learn the Key to Prevailing Prayer

Rees Howells was a man uniquely taught of God who found the key to prevailing prayer, became the channel of a mighty revival in Africa, was taught the principles of divine healing and progressed even further in faith until world events were affected by his prayers.

Trade paper ISBN: 978-0-87508-188-5